Endocrinology Research and Clinical Developments

nova
Medicine & Health
New York

Endocrinology Research and Clinical Developments

Natural Products for Treatment of Metabolic Syndrome
Ajmer Singh Grewal, PhD (Editors)
Ashwani Kumar Dhingra, PhD (Editors)
2022. ISBN: 979-8-88697-152-1 (Hardcover)
2022. ISBN: 979-8-88697-233-7 (eBook)

A Clinical Guide to Thyroidectomies
Anand Mishra (Editor)
2022. ISBN: 978-1-68507-814-0 (Hardcover)
2022. ISBN: 979-8-88697-033-3 (eBook)

Polycystic Ovary Syndrome: Causes, Diagnosis and Management
Katherine Webb (Editor)
2021. ISBN: 978-1-53619-527-9 (Softcover)
2021. ISBN: 978-1-53619-586-6 (eBook)

Diabetes and Diabetic Complications: Current Status and Future Perspectives
Randhir Singh Dahiya (Editor)
Thakur Gurjeet Singh (Editor)
2021. ISBN: 978-1-53619-177-6 (Hardcover)
2021. ISBN: 978-1-53619-453-1 (eBook)

Gestational Diabetes: From Diagnosis to Treatment
Hasan Aydin (Editor)
2020. ISBN: 978-1-53618-335-1 (Hardcover)
2020. ISBN: 978-1-53618-578-2 (eBook)

More information about this series can be found at
https://novapublishers.com/product-category/series/endocrinology-research-and-clinical-developments/

David Aebisher
Editor

The Biochemical Guide to Hormones

nova
Medicine & Health
New York

https://doi.org/10.52305/AEZF7790

Library of Congress Cataloging-in-Publication Data

ISBN: 979-8-88697-492-8

Published by Nova Science Publishers, Inc. † New York

Contents

Preface

This book aims to provide scientific information about hormones. Hormones are chemical compounds that transmit specific information between organs and thus regulate the body's work. As a group of biologically active signaling molecules, it belongs to the four main groups of organic chemical compounds. The written chapters 36 present the characteristics of exemplary hormones. The prepared monograph is a description of the most popular hormones. In book we can read about the biochemical pathways of adrenaline, adrenocorticotropic hormone (ACTH), aldosterone, antidiuretic hormone (vasopressin), cholecystokinin, corticosteroid, corticotropin releasing hormone (CRH), Cortisol, endocrine disorders, endocrine system, Epinephrine, Erythropoietin, Estrogen, Follicle-stimulatg hormone (FSH), Ghrelin, Glucagon, Gonadotropin releasing hormone (GnRH), growth hormone (GH), Growth hormone releasing hormone (GHRH), hepcidin, human chorionic gonadotropin-β, Humoral factors, Importance of a correct hormonal balance for the psychological well-being of women, Insulin, Insulin-like growth factor (IGF), luteinizing hormone (LH), insulin, oxytocin, parathyroid hormone (PTH), progesterone, prolactinThyroid-stimulating hormone (TSH), Serotonin, thyroid hormone, thyrotropin releasing hormone (TRH) and prolactin.

Chapter 1

Analogs of Insulin

Cezary Buszta, Dorota Bartusik-Aebisher*
and David Aebisher
Medical College of The University of Rzeszów, Rzeszów, Poland

Abstract

Diabetes mellitus is a disease of civilization that affects more and more people. The cause of diabetes is the development of humanity, i.e., urbanization and ensuring a better and better life. People are increasingly choosing a sedentary lifestyle, often driven by higher factors. Insulin replacement therapy is necessary for many patients suffering from this disease. The market today uses more sophisticated methods that rely on insulin analogues to alter the time it takes for insulin to be absorbed by cells with the need for glucose. Diabetes has long been diagnosed, but much is not known yet because treatment does not completely eliminate the disease. This creates a great challenge for the future, including in molecular diagnostics, where defective, mutated and disease-determining genes can be examined.

Keywords: insulin, hormone, diabetes, glargine, Langerhans cells, obesity, pancreatic

Diabetes affects many people in the world. From year to year, more and more patients with this serious disease are increasing. Already nearly 25.4 million Americans have type 2 diabetes. The reason for the reduction in insulin levels

---

* Corresponding Author's Email: dbartusikaebisher@ur.edu.pl.

In: The Biochemical Guide to Hormones
Editor: David Aebisher
ISBN: 979-8-88697-492-8

in this disease is the lack or reduction in the synthesis of pancreatic Langerhans cells, also known as β cells. Insulin replacement therapy is necessary for many patients suffering from this disease. After the discovery of insulin in the 1920s, steps were taken to prolong the activity of this protein. Including it was zinc but also other preparations, i.e., NPH (neutral protamin Hagedorn) (Mathieu et al., 2017). In contrast, these substances were not found to be effective because their duration of action was too short or too long, and they were ultimately not introduced into insulin replacement therapy between meals or with food consumption. The market today uses more sophisticated methods that rely on insulin analogues to alter the time it takes for insulin to be absorbed by cells with the need for glucose. This is to control its concentration throughout the day, which results in the normalization of the monosaccharide content in the circulating blood. The mentioned analogs are glargine and detemir, which have a longer absorption time than NPH and human insulin, so they can better control blood sugar levels (Mathieu et al., 2017).

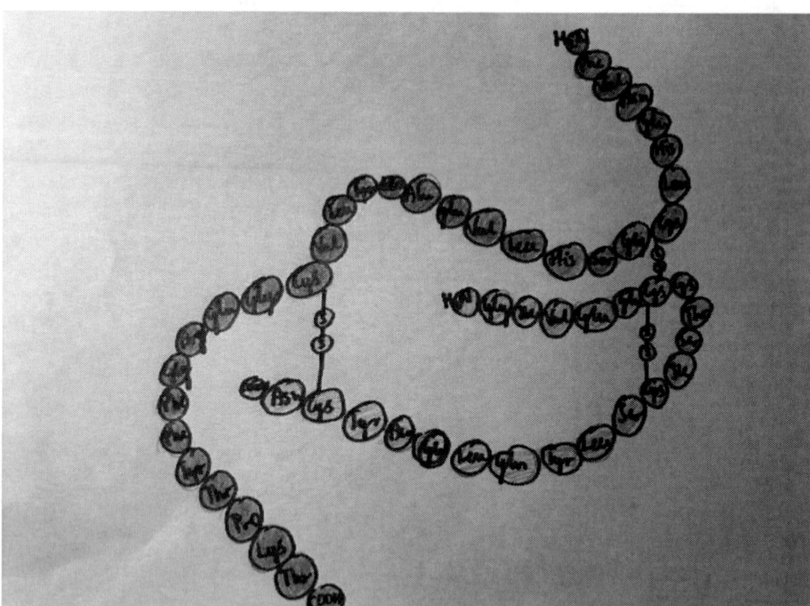

Figure 1. The quaternary structure of human insulin. It consists of two chains, A and B, connected by disulfide bridges, stabilizing the protein structure. [Own study].

Glargine was the first insulin analog created by recombinant DNA technology. Asparagine was replaced with glycine and arginine residues were added to the B-chain at the C-terminus. Arginine plays a key role as it causes all injected substance to be absorbed later, resulting in higher levels of the hormone and more efficient transport of sugar to the cells. In addition, it inhibits proteolysis and lipolysis, i.e., it is anti-catabolic. Studies have shown that insulin glargine is a repressor on glucose synthesis and is more effective than the administered glucose uptake stimulators. Measurement of the concentration of the analog is difficult because it is structurally similar to the actual hormone and is costly. The technique used to measure the concentration of glargine is mass spectrometry. Immunoassays detect cross-reactivity between both substances, so that the appropriate concentration of the analog can be administered for the most effective therapy (Posner et al., 2016).

It is a substance that reduces the release of glucose from the liver. The consequence is not only a reduction in blood glucose levels, but also a decrease in insulin sensitivity. The use of this preparation makes a lot of sense because it facilitates the functioning of the body in the case of a hormone deficiency, produced in the diseased pancreas. What's more, it reduces the risk of coronary heart disease, which can often appear as a side effect of long-term diabetes (Santoleri et al., 2019).

The cause of diabetes is the development of humanity, i.e., urbanization and ensuring a better and better life. People are increasingly choosing a sedentary lifestyle, often driven by higher factors. In a country like China, the nutritional trend has changed, causing various diseases such as diabetes. Research shows that changing your daily habits to healthier ones reduces the risk of developing cysticerculosis. disease by 28.5%. The problem with glucose intolerance also applies to pregnant women. There is talk of gestational diabetes. A 10-year study showed that such women had a 70% higher chance of developing pancreatic disease, which could also have an impact on the child's health, e.g., metabolism, hormonal imbalance, etc. Child malnutrition, caused mainly by the mother's poor diet, caused increased risk of cardiometabolic disease. In a test on poorly fed animals, problems with pancreatic beta-cell dysfunction were much more common (Tokarz et al., 2018). It concerns type 1 and type 2 diabetes. It is related to the apoptosis of cells that synthesize insulin. The problem also applies to diseases such as obesity or insulin sensitivity. The reduction in the weight of the pancreas is 40% to 65%. Evidence of the dysfunction of this gland is the secretion of proinsulin and amyloid fibrils into the bloodstream. The latter are toxic to the sites of their secretion. They cause sudden apoptosis. As their concentration increases, so does the number of cells killed, so blood levels may indicate the severity of the disease (Tokarz et al., 2018).

As mentioned in the case of global problems, you have to start with yourself, i.e., change your lifestyle. Adequate diet and exercise reduce the risk of cardiovascular disease and lead to weight loss. Obesity often correlates with diabetes. Therapy can also be metroformin, which literally rests the cells that build the damaged organ.

Increased blood lipids and muscle lipids impair insulin function. This reduces glucose uptake. An excess of free fatty acids increases insulin resistance, i.e., cells are less susceptible to the action of the pancreatic hormone. However, the intake of LDL-rich food and the synthesis of ApoB (Apolipoprotein B – builds LDL acids) viciously lead to atherogenic dyslipidemia. Methods for the reduction of comorbidities of diabetes include: methods of bariatric surgery, where e.g., gastroplasty is performed. The goal is to lose weight and reduce this risk factor, which is defined as one of the leading causes of pancreatic disease (Titchenel et al. 2017).

Adipose tissue produces many hormones and mediators, e.g., leptin, NEFA (NMDA receptor antagonist) and adiponectin. Increased intracellular concentration of NEFA competes with glucose, which inhibits pyruvate dehydrogenase processes. This results in the failure of glucose to enter the Krebs cycle and the accumulation of glucose-6-phosphate, which inhibits the cellular uptake of glucose. Insulin activation decreases and blood sugar increases (Titchenel et al., 2017).

Diabetes mellitus is a disease of civilization that affects more and more people. Man has changed his thinking by focusing on achievements and reducing self-perception, e.g., looking at how he eats. The consequences are systemic disorders, leading to faster death. Pancreatic disease is associated with the degeneration of many organs, i.e., heart, liver and kidneys. Medicines and various health aids have been developed to reduce the effects of the disease and prolong life.

Sometimes it is possible to get sick not of your own free will, e.g., pregnant women, whose risk of falling ill increases significantly. However, the vast majority of it depends a lot on genetic factors and the choices of everyday life. Adipose tissue plays a large role in the formation of diabetes, which is evidence that the pancreas works with tissues, differing in formation during gastrulation.

Diabetes has long been diagnosed, but much is not known yet because treatment does not completely eliminate the disease. This creates a great challenge for the future, including in molecular diagnostics, where defective, mutated and disease-determining genes can be examined. Pancreatic β cells have a nucleus containing cellular DNA, which is the main source of mutation.

Knowledge about the protein genes coding for proteins, i.e., insulin, allows us to identify possible defects and find a way to treat a very troublesome disease – diabetes.

References

Mathieu C, Gillard P, Benhalima K. Insulin analogues in type 1 diabetes mellitus: Getting better all the time. *Nat Rev Endocrinol*, 2017; 13(7):385-399.

Posner BI. Insulin Signalling: The Inside Story. *Can J Diabetes*, 2017 Feb; 41(1):108-113.

Santoleri D, Titchenell PM. Resolving the Paradox of Hepatic Insulin Resistance. *Cell Mol Gastroenterol Hepatol,* 2019; 7(2):447-456.

Titchenell PM, Lazar MA, Birnbaum MJ. Unraveling the Regulation of Hepatic Metabolism by Insulin. *Trends Endocrinol Metab*, 2017; 28(7):497-505.

Tokarz VL, MacDonald PE, Klip A. The cell biology of systemic insulin function. *J Cell Biol,* 2018; 217(7):2273-2289.

Chapter 2

Insulin-Like Growth Factor (IGF)

Katarzyna Piekarz, Dorota Bartusik-Aebisher[*]
and David Aebisher
Medical College of The University of Rzeszów, Rzeszów, Poland

Abstract

Insulin-like growth factor (IGF) is a peptide hormone that has a significant impact on the growth and development of the body. Its concentration depends on age, gender, insulin levels and nutritional status. In the human body throughout life, the processes of synthesis of building components take place, the replacement of worn-out cells and the reconstruction of tissues caused by damage of various origins takes place, which makes the presence of this ligand in the blood plasma necessary throughout life. The most disturbing and at the same time giving therapeutic hope is the influence of IGF on the pathological proliferation of cells manifested in neoplasms. The high activity of this hormone can lead to the development of the disease. However, knowing the structure of IGF and its receptors well, attempts are made to develop substances that act as inhibitors of IGF-IR receptors in tissues and prevent cells from multiplying in pathological conditions.

Keywords: IGF-I, Insulin-like growth factor (IGF), growth hormone (GH), Insulin receptors

---

[*] Corresponding Author's Email: dbartusikaebisher@ur.edu.pl.

In: The Biochemical Guide to Hormones
Editor: David Aebisher
ISBN: 979-8-88697-492-8

Insulin-like growth factor (IGF) is a peptide hormone that is produced in the liver. Its structure is similar to that of insulin and therefore it has an affinity for its receptors. It comes in two forms: IGF-1, otherwise known as somatomedin C, and IGF-2. It is essential for the proper growth and development of tissues. It keeps the concentration of calcium, magnesium and potassium in the body at a constant level. Its effect is cell proliferation and changes in glucose metabolism. It has neurosecretory and cardioprotective effects. In addition, it regulates mitogenic functions. IFG is stimulated by growth hormone (GH). Its concentration depends on age, gender, insulin levels and nutritional status. The highest concentration is observed during fetal life and intensive growth, where it has a significant effect. During childhood, higher concentrations are observed in girls than in boys. Its concentration decreases with age – after 40 years of age. Premature decline in IGF levels below normal leads to many abnormalities, such as growth disorders in children (dwarfism) and adults, lipid disorders, decreased muscle mass, decreased bone density, malnutrition, kidney and liver diseases. Elevated levels of this hormone occur during pregnancy (IGF-1 only), and pathological growth may manifest itself as gigantism and acromegaly. In the vascular bed, a significant proportion of IGF is bound to carrier proteins, which increases its plasma half-life (Adamek et al., 2018).

IGF-I is a polypeptide chain of 70 amino acids with a molecular weight of 7.6 kDa. In its structure, it has three disulfide bridges between amino acids 6 and 48, 18 and 61, and 47 and 52. Their presence causes that IGF-I has a tertiary structure, which enables connection with a specific receptor for IGF-I. Its affinity for the receptor is 100 times higher than for insulin. IGF-II is similar in structure to IGF-I, however, the polypeptide chain that builds its molecule is more than twice as large and amounts to 180 amino acids (Gusscott et al., 2019).

IGF-I and IGF-II act on IGF-I receptors (IGF-IR) – the tyrosine kinase receptor. In addition, it can additionally bind to the IGF-II receptor, known as the cation-independent mannose-6-phosphate receptor. The structure of IGF-IR consists of two α chains and two β chains connected by disulphide bridges. There is a binding site for the insulin-like factor IGF-I on the α subunit. Activation of the IGF-IR receptor leads to a conformational change in the β subunits. This allows for the attachment of additional signaling molecules. The formation of an active receptor causes numerous signaling cascades, thanks to which they have a real impact on the regulation of various activities, e.g., cell proliferation. IGF-I acts as a hormone. It is produced in the liver and then transported to target tissues. Synthesis and secretion also take place outside the liver, where IGF-I acts locally in a paracrine fashion (Kraemer et al., 2020).

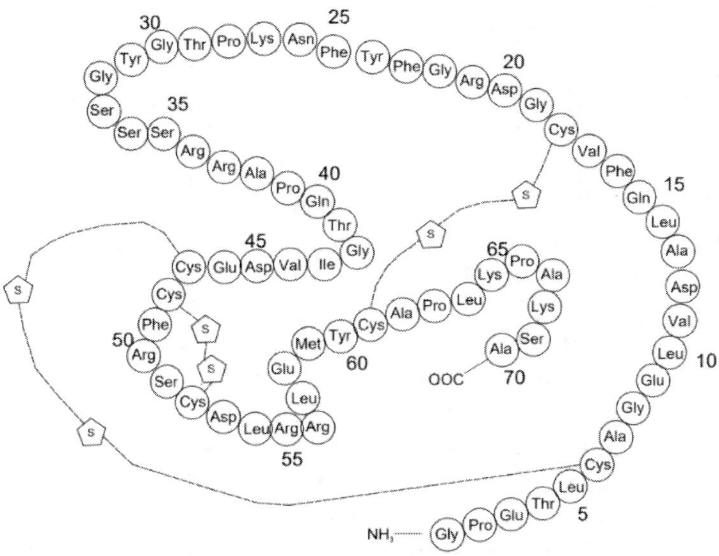

Figure 1. Structure of human insulin-like growth factor. The illustration shows the primary structure showing the disulfide bridges.

Insulin receptors (INSR) are present in target tissues sensitive to the action of this hormone: liver, muscles and adipose tissue. They work by controlling anabolism and glucose homeostasis. These receptors have a high affinity for insulin, but also to a lesser extent for IGF. The concentration of insulin in the blood is precisely controlled and secreted from the β cells of the pancreas for circulation in response to the increase in blood glucose. The concentration of IGF-I IGF-II is regulated by growth hormone (GH), but in the case of IGF-II the control is weak and these ligands are not stored after synthesis. It can therefore be assumed that disturbances in the synthesis leading to a change in IGF concentration may affect the proper functioning of INSR receptors (Kraemer et al., 2020).

Abnormal regulation of IGF-I and IGF-IR expression may lead to tumor development. This is because in a state of homeostasis IGF is responsible for the regulation of proper proliferation and the life cycle of the cell. The high bioactivity of IGF-I will stimulate oncogenesis in some tissues of the human body and be involved in the development of colon, breast, thyroid and prostate cancer. The therapeutic strategy used in the fight against cancer is the inhibition of IGF receptors. One of the substances is the αIR3 antibody, which inhibited the growth of neoplastic cells in the breasts in vitro. However, there are concerns about the negative impact of this inhibitor on tissue IGF-IR receptors and the interaction of INSRs necessary for the proper functioning of the human body. Other strategies rely on a molecular approach, anti-IGF-IR antibodies, small molecule tyrosine kinase inhibitors (TKIs), IGF-I / II neutralizing antibodies and IGF TRAP ligands. They are at the stage of pre-clinical and clinical trials. However, I hope to discover an effective drug in the treatment of neoplastic changes (Poreba et al., 2020).

Clinical studies have shown that a complete or partial deletion of the IGF-I or IGF-IR gene causes mental retardation and growth. In addition to the above-mentioned increased risk of chronic cancer incidence, a high concentration of IGF-I increases bone fragility, where it is involved in their development in the correct amount. Other diseases that depend on the concentration of insulin-like growth factor are gigantism, acromegaly and dwarfism. The ignition mechanism of IGF deviations from the norm, and thus the incidence of these diseases, is overproduction in the case of gigantism and acromegaly, and deficiency in the case of growth hormone (GH) dwarfism. Fluctuations in IGF concentration also increase the risk of insulin resistance in type II diabetes, thyroid diseases such as Graves' disease and skin diseases: psoriasis and acne (Takahashi et al., 2017). Insulin-like growth factor (IGF) is a peptide hormone that has a significant impact on the growth and development of the body. The resulting regularity is the observation of the highest concentration of this hormone in prenatal life and in adolescence, when the body grows intensively. In the human body throughout life, the processes of synthesis of building components take place, the replacement of worn-out cells and the reconstruction of tissues caused by damage of various origins takes place, which makes the presence of this ligand in the blood plasma necessary throughout life. Structure similar to insulin gives great therapeutic potential, but also carries the risk of various types of disorders caused by changes in the concentration of this hormone. The production and secretion of IGF is growth hormone (GH) dependent, so the cascade of disorders caused by abnormal IGF levels may have its origins in the pituitary gland and even in the hypothalamus. Fluctuations in IGF concentration are dangerous because they can lead to many diseases related to the development and growth of the human body, such as dwarfism, gigantism, acromegaly or bone fragility, but also can lead to thyroid and skin diseases. The most disturbing and at the same time giving therapeutic hope is the influence of IGF on the pathological proliferation of cells manifested in neoplasms. The high activity of this hormone can lead to the development of the disease. However, knowing the structure of IGF and its receptors well, attempts are made to develop substances that act as inhibitors of IGF-IR receptors in tissues and prevent cells from multiplying in pathological conditions.

References

Adamek A, Kasprzak A. Insulin-Like Growth Factor (IGF) System in Liver Diseases. *Int J Mol Sci,* 2018; 19(5):1308.

Gusscott S, Tamiro F, Giambra V, Weng AP. Insulin-like growth factor (IGF) signaling in T-cell acute lymphoblastic leukemia. *Adv Biol Regul,* 2019; 74:100652.

Kraemer WJ, Ratamess NA, Hymer WC, Nindl BC, Fragala MS. Growth Hormone(s), Testosterone, Insulin-Like Growth Factors, and Cortisol: Roles and Integration for Cellular Development and Growth with Exercise. *Front Endocrinol*, (Lausanne). 2020; 11:33.

Poreba E, Durzynska J. Nuclear localization and actions of the insulin-like growth factor 1 (IGF-1) system components: Transcriptional regulation and DNA damage response. *Mutat Res Rev Mutat Res,* 2020; 784:108307.

Takahashi Y. The Role of Growth Hormone and Insulin-Like Growth Factor-I in the Liver. *Int J Mol Sci,* 2017; 18(7):1447.

Chapter 3

Oxytocin

Oliwia Wójcik, Sylwia Lepak, Dorota Bartusik-Aebisher* and David Aebisher
Medical College of The University of Rzeszów, Rzeszów, Poland

Abstract

Oxytocin is a very important protein that is important in many areas of human physiology. There is a lot of research on its applications, but a large part is not yet confirmed due to too few people being tested. Undeniably, however, oxytocin can be assigned a number of roles in experiencing emotions and generating personality traits. It is clear from many studies that increased activity of this hormone moderates or reverses the effects of abused drugs. Unfortunately, there is still no exact explanation for the changes in neuroplasticity. It plays an important role in nutritional processes. This hormone, in the future, may be a salvation for people with diseases such as autism, Alzheimer's disease or bulimia. Performing more tests and introducing it as a drug (in other conditions than used so far) has a chance to improve the quality of life of many people.

Keywords: oxytocin, hormone, Alzheimer's disease, nonapeptide, anorexigenic, mitogenically

Oxytocin is a 9 amino acid peptide hormone that commonly functions as a neurotransmitter. The name of the hormone comes from the Greek language and means "quick labor," which is closely related to the role of oxytocin. One

* Corresponding Author's Email: dbartusikaebisher@ur.edu.pl.

In: The Biochemical Guide to Hormones
Editor: David Aebisher
ISBN: 979-8-88697-492-8

of its main functions is to induce labor in the final stages, stimulating uterine contractions, resulting in the displacement of the child from the woman's genital tract. Oxytocin is synthesized in the paraventricular nucleus of the hypothalamus, from where it is transported to the posterior pituitary gland, where it is stored (Carter et al., 2020).

Further regulation of secretion depends on the level of estrogens (they increase production) and progesterone (inhibit production), or on mechanical stimulation of the nipples, receptors of the vaginal walls and cervix. Many other oxytocin-dependent mechanisms influencing the functioning of the digestive system, emotional aspects, or nervous system dysfunctions leading to mental disorders were also investigated. Oxytocin was the first hormone that could be obtained synthetically. The result obtained in this way is used to speed up the labor. After giving birth, it is designed to reduce bleeding. It has also been proven to be a substance that causes mutual attachment to another person. It is associated with trust and building relationships. When two people are brought together, it makes them more attractive to each other. This hormone has an impact on achieving orgasm in women and erection in men. It also contributes to the occurrence of a phenomenon known as the maternal instinct. There is a lot of research on the treatment of mental disorders with oxytocin, which psychiatrists have high hopes for (Carter et al., 2020).

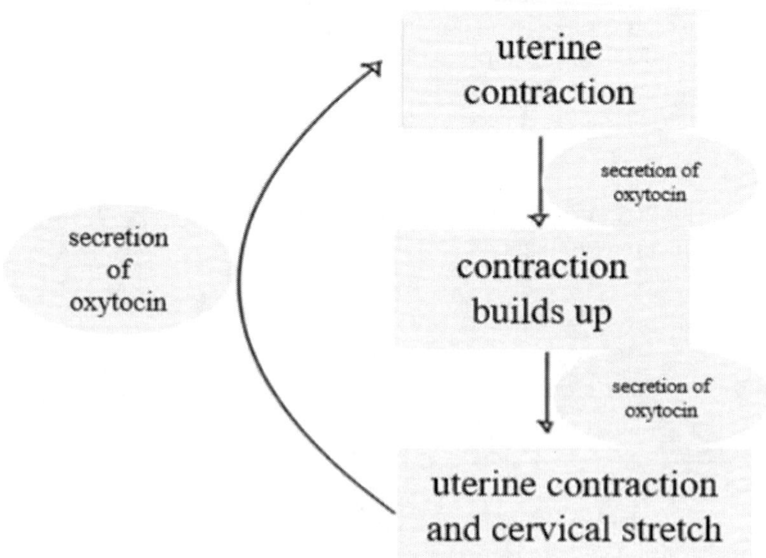

Figure 1. The action of oxytocin on the uterus.

Oxytocin stimulates uterine contractions by activating receptor-bound sodium channels and releasing calcium from the endoplasmic reticulum. Oxytocin binds to the receptor and is influenced by a voltage- or endocrine-regulated secondary messenger on the cell membrane of the muscle fiber as well as by extracellular calcium influx. Oxytocin increases the production of inositol 1,4,5-triphosphate and mobilizes the release of inositol 5-triphosphate by the endoplasmic and sarcoplasmic reticulum. Moreover, oxytocin contributes to the generation of internal currents by cells through non-selective, receptor-dependent cation channels. They cause the depolarization of cell membranes, generating action potentials and muscle contractions. In vitro experiments with human uterine myocytes are derived from the period when pregnancy signals the effect of oxytocin on uterine contractions by depolarizing the cell membrane, but without affecting the interaction of muscle fibers through gap junctions, indicating uterine contraction and myocyte coordination. The mechanism of activity is different. At present, the role of secondary messengers such as cAMP and cGMP is unknown. In vitro studies have shown that cAMP is involved in the exponential increase in the number of amniotic oxytocin receptors during pregnancy in rabbits. Oxytocin also increases the activity of mitogenically activated kinases through the G protein. It increases the activity of alanine aminotransferase and phospholipase C by binding the oxytocin receptor to the G-alpha q and G-alpha 11 chains of the protein attached (Marlin et al., 2017).

The structures of oxytocin and vasopressin are very similar to each other. They are of the same origin and are made of 2,500 pairs of nucleotides. The gene encoding oxytocin consists of 3 exons and 2 introns and is located on the 20th chromosome. The nine amino acids that make up oxytocin are cysteine, tyrosine, isoleucine, glutamine, asparagine, cysteine, proline, leucine, and glycine, respectively. This hormone is transported from the paraventricular nucleus of the hypothalamus to the posterior pituitary gland. The secretion of oxytocin is stimulated by estrogens and inhibited by progesterone. Secretion occurs when the nipples are irritated, thereby producing milk. Another stimulant is the action on the receptors of the vaginal walls and cervix. It accelerates the labor and constricts the blood vessels in the uterine wall, preventing bleeding after expulsion of the placenta. It influences the feeling of emotions in mammals, such as jealousy, trust, submission, and the ability to cooperate (Marlin et al., 2017).

The synthesis of oxytocin begins with the condensation of N-carbobenzoxy-S-benzyl-L-cysteinyl-L-tyrosine and L-isoleucyl-L-glutaminyl-L-asparaginyl-S-benzyl-L-cysteinyl-L-prolyl-L-leucylglycinamide, leading to the formation of a nonapeptide. This process is followed by reduction in the presence of sodium in ammonia solution and oxidation to form the nonapeptide sulfhydryl. L-isoleucyl-L-glutaminyl-L-asparaginyl-S-benzyl-L-cysteinyl-L-prolyl-L-leucylglycinamide is formed by the synthesis of S-benzyl-L-cysteinyl-L-prolyl-L-leucylglycinamide from toxyl-L -isoleucyl-L-glutaminyl-L-asparagine, which precedes removal of the toxyl group from the condensation product. The biologically active synthetic material obtained in the presented manner is purified and laboratory compared with the naturally occurring oxytocin (Jones et al., 2017).

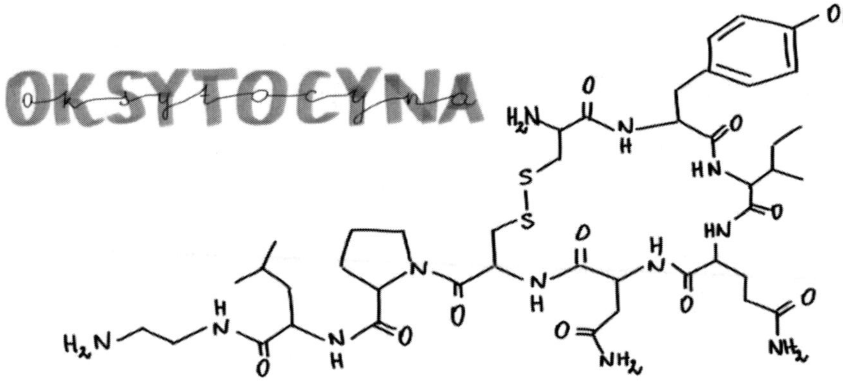

Figure 2. Oxytocin.

Scientists have been looking at oxytocin as a potential therapeutic option for people with multiple neurological diseases for many years. This hormone is best known for its role in the birth process, and it also has anxiolytic properties, influences the processes of addiction, aggression, and learning and remembering. Within the amygdala, oxytocin reduces anxiety and inhibits stress reactions, and within the lateral septum, it is involved in pro-social behavior, including social preferences.

Social anxiety is a constant fear of many relationship situations in society. The causes of this disease are multifactorial and include genetics, neurobiology, fetal and postpartum environment. The conducted research shows a relationship between anxiety and alleles of the oxytocin receptor gene. Animal studies show that the administration of oxytocin stimulates and accelerates the formation of pairs. Central administration of this hormone to rats improves their social memory, and an oxytocin receptor antagonist blocks this type of memory. It was found that oxytocin can alter stress neural connectivity and cause social cohesion after the stressor that usually causes distraction. Studies conducted on macaques confirmed that after administration of oxytocin, they made more pro-social choices (shared juice). Restricting eye contact is a common symptom of mental illness, including social phobia and autism. Excessive analysis of social situations perceived as threatening is part of social anxiety. Experience shows that oxytocin prolongs eye contact and eases social alertness. Administering it reduces the level of cortisol that is released in response to stress. Research focuses mainly on the amygdala as it is overactive in times of danger. Oxytocin inhibits the neurons in the amygdala from attaching to other fear structures. It normalizes the pathways responsible for the feeling of anxiety. The studies mainly used the intranasal route of administration as oxytocin does not cross the blood-brain barrier and oral and intravenous administration is ineffective (Jones et al., 2017).

Methamphetamine is a highly addictive stimulant. The short-term effects of taking it are: an increase in energy levels, alertness, and excitement. Long-term use causes cardiovascular disorders. Animal studies have been conducted on the effects of oxytocin on addiction to this substance. Oxytocin was investigated to influence the induction but not the expression of methamphetamine-induced CPP. This hormone has also been shown to reduce rats' motivation to search for drugs. In men addicted to alcohol, the immunoreactivity of OXT peptides was reduced compared to the control group. Overall, exposure to drugs and alcohol causes compensatory neuroadaptive changes in the endogenous OXT system in areas of the brain particularly involved in the addiction process. Dysfunctional social behaviors related to reward and stress are the result of impaired functioning of this system in the brain. Administration of oxytocin may have benefits in restoring behavior by compensating for abnormalities in the brain caused by prolonged exposure to alcohol or drugs. (Yoon et al., 2020).

Oxytocin also plays a role in the relationship between psychosocial and digestive behavior. Changes in the paraventricular nucleus, one of the main production sites of oxytocin, increase the amount of food consumed. Administration of oxytocin intraperitoneally or intracerebroventrically results in a reduction in these amounts. It has been shown that this hormone is an indirect mediator of the action of leptin and that it activates propiomelanocortin neurons – elements of the anorexigenic system. In obese subjects, intranasal administration of oxytocin has been found to reduce food intake. Unfortunately, more studies are needed on larger groups to confirm these results. The latest results indicate a deficiency of oxytocin in people with anorexia nervosa. In the experiment on the amount of calories consumed in people with anorexia and bulimia, after administering one dose of oxytocin, a decrease in food consumption occurred only in people with bulimia. In subsequent tests, it was proved that intranasal administration of oxytocin, 4 times a day, resulted in a weight loss of about 9 kg among the test group. Genetic data show, however, that the influence of this hormone depends on the possessed alleles by the tested person (Yamasue et al., 2018).

Oxytocin is a very important protein that is important in many areas of human physiology. There is a lot of research on its applications, but a large part is not yet confirmed due to too few people being tested. Understanding the structure and exact mode of action of oxytocin allowed scientists not only to analyze the processes taking place with its participation. Certainly, a promising step turned out to be the knowledge that allows for the synthesis of oxytocin in a synthetic manner in laboratory conditions. This ability makes it possible to use oxytocin therapy in numerous disorders, taking into account the multitude of processes affected by this hormone. During the isolation of structures, analogies in the structure between oxytocin and vasopressin, which are linked, among others, by the same number of nucleotides, were also noticed. The commonly recognized role of the described nonapeptide is to influence the female reproductive system and the action of childbirth. Undeniably, however, oxytocin can be assigned a number of roles in experiencing emotions and generating personality traits. This is also related to its importance in psychology or psychiatry.

It is clear from many studies that increased activity of this hormone moderates or reverses the effects of abused drugs. Exogenous administration of oxytocin reduces the need for a stimulant. Unfortunately, there is still no exact explanation for the changes in neuroplasticity. It plays an important role in nutritional processes. In stressful situations, it reduces mental discomfort and helps in coping with anxiety in such circumstances. This hormone, in the future, may be a salvation for people with diseases such as autism, Alzheimer's disease or bulimia. Performing more tests and introducing it as a drug (in other conditions than used so far) has a chance to improve the quality of life of many people.

References

Carter C S, Kenkel W M, MacLean E L, Wilson S R, Perkeybile A M, Yee J R, Ferris C F, Nazarloo H P, Porges S W, Davis J M, Connelly J J, Kingsbury M A. Is Oxytocin "Nature's Medicine"? *Pharmacol. Rev*. 2020 Oct;72(4):829-861.

Jones C, Barrera I, Brothers S, Ring R, Wahlestedt C. Oxytocin and social functioning. *Dialogues Clin. Neurosci*. 2017 Jun;19(2):193-201.

Marlin B J, Froemke R C. Oxytocin modulation of neural circuits for social behavior. *Dev. Neurobiol.* 2017 Feb;77(2):169-189.

Yamasue H, Domes G. Oxytocin and Autism Spectrum Disorders. *Curr. Top. Behav. Neurosci.* 2018;35:449-465.

Yoon S, Kim Y K. The Role of the Oxytocin System in Anxiety Disorders. *Adv. Exp. Med. Biol.* 2020;1191:103-120.

Chapter 4

Human Chorionic Gonadotropin-β

Marcin Skowronek, Dorota Bartusik-Aebisher*
and David Aebisher
Medical College of The University of Rzeszów, Rzeszów, Poland

Abstract

Human Chorionic Gonadotrophin (hCG) is the first hormone to be included in the group of pregnancy hormones as early as 1928. Many recent studies on human chorionic gonadotropin hCG prove that this hormone plays an essential role in the correct implantation of the fetus and the further development of pregnancy. It is presumed that, as it is during pregnancy, hCG acts as a regulator of cell formation and apoptosis, contributing to the development of immune tolerance of the mother's organism to the fetus and tumor antigens. During tumor development, hCG may show various counter-positive effects. A thorough understanding of the function of the chorionic gonadotropin can lead to many modern medical applications of this hormone. Understanding the hCG-mediated pathways should result in the future designation of new diagnostic and therapeutic strategies for both pregnancy and neoplastic disease.

Keywords: human chorionic gonadotrophin (hCG), follicle stimulating hormone (FSH), Hormones Lutropin (LH), protein kinase C (PKC)

---

* Corresponding Author's Email: dbartusikaebisher@ur.edu.pl.

In: The Biochemical Guide to Hormones
Editor: David Aebisher
ISBN: 979-8-88697-492-8

Human Chorionic Gonadotrophin (hCG) is a hormone of the glycoprotein family, which also includes the anterior pituitary hormones lutropin (LH), follicle stimulating hormone (FSH) and thyrotropin (TSH), produced by trophoblast cells during pregnancy. hCG is the first hormone to be included in the group of pregnancy hormones as early as 1928. It is also considered one of the most important hormones controlling the development and course of pregnancy. Physiologically, it affects the embryo implantation, angiogenesis and chorionic villus development, and disturbances in the secretion of this hormone may indicate abnormalities during pregnancy or lead to serious complications. hCG is made up of two non-covalent linked subunits: alpha (α) and beta (β), making it a heterodimer. The first one is common to the gonadotropin family, while the second one determines the specificity of the whole hormone. The structure of the beta subunit is shown in Figure 1. They are synthesized independently of each other and controlled by various transcription factors (Gonzalez et al., 2017).

The expression mechanism of human chorionic gonadotropin is not fully known, and research indicates that epigenetic factors are also important in the synthesis of this hormone, especially the beta subunit. hCG can also be used as a marker. Determination of the presence of the hormone in blood or urine is used in pregnancy tests, moreover, chorionic gonadotropin has been detected in many tumors of various origins. So far, the role of hCG in carcinogenesis has not been elucidated. This hormone is believed to promote the development, growth and metastasis of tumors (Gonzalez et al., 2017).

Human Chorionic Gonadotrophin (hCG) is a hormone that is produced and secreted at a very early stage of embryonic development. In humans, the expression of the hCG gene occurs at the stage of two blastomers, and the detection of this protein is possible at the stage of the blastocyst. Chorionic gonadotrophin can affect pregnancy both directly and indirectly. The direct action of hCG is shown by the regulation of the functions of the cells of the womb lining (endometrium), including the cells of the glandular epithelium, lining and connective tissue. These cells contain an hCG-sensitive receptor. Under the influence of the hormone, the uterine glands become swollen and twisted during pregnancy, and their secretory function increases. The synthesis of smooth muscle actin in the stromal fibroblasts of the uterine mucosa is also stimulated. These changes significantly affect the temporal transformation, causing the formation of temporal tissue responsible for the protection and nourishment of the implanting embryo (Hendriks et al., 2020).

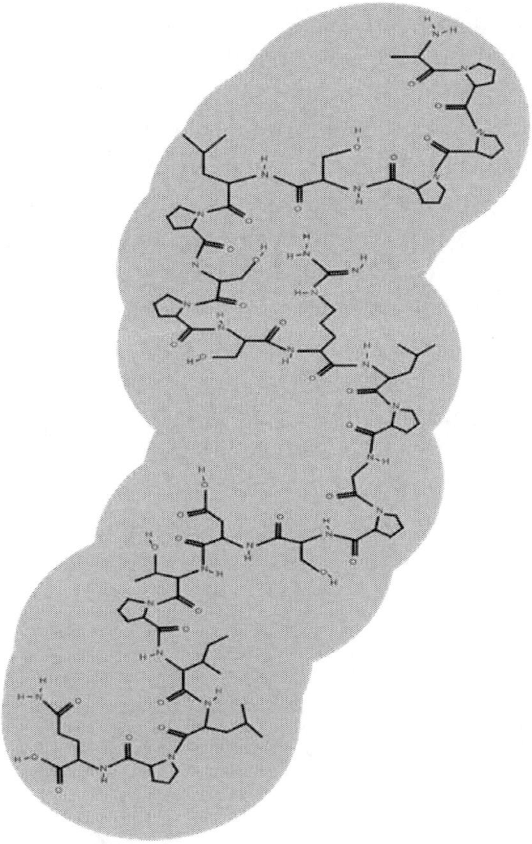

Figure 1. Human chorionic gonadotropin (hCG), beta subunit (β-hCG). [Own study].

Chorionic gonadotropin determines the proper implantation and, subsequently, the success of pregnancy development by regulating the temporal transformation and influencing the process of apoptosis, the formation of blood vessels (angiogenesis) and protection against the maternal immune system. One of the most important phenomena leading to the exfoliation of the endometrium during menstrual periods is suicide cell death, or apoptosis. Under the influence of hCG, the apoptotic proteins Bcl-2 and Bax are inhibited. This suppresses the regression of the stromal cells of the uterine mucosa and prevents its transition to the exfoliative (menstrual) phase (Hendriks et al., 2019).

The process of formation of new blood vessels during the implantation period is an important process also regulated by the chorionic gonadotropin.

During pregnancy, the need for blood and its supply to the placenta increases, which results in the remodeling of blood vessels. hCG causes the expansion and permeability of the blood vessel wall, and is responsible for the activation of protein kinase C (PKC), which stimulates the formation of new blood vessels in the endometrium. One of the many processes taking place during implantation is an inflammatory reaction along with the immune response of the mother's body, which is reduced by the chorionic gonadotropin. This hormone inhibits the activity of T lymphocytes and the secretion of pro-inflammatory cytokines by endometrial cells (Schüler-Toprak et al., 2017).

The determination of the hCG hormone is an extremely important factor in the biochemical diagnosis of a proper pregnancy. The chorionic gonadotropin produced by the trophoblast is the basis of pregnancy immunological tests. In the blood serum, hCG is detectable on the 9th to 11th day after ovulation sewing of LH concentration, i.e., on the 8th day after ovulation, and also on the first day after embryo implantation. The level of hCG, especially beta-hCG, is a very diagnostic element in complications of early pregnancy. Factors to consider when a pregnancy abnormality is suspected include:

- ectopic pregnancy;
- death of pregnancy;
- empty fetal egg;
- mate a bunny.

It should be noted that the diagnostic process of β-hCG is a dynamic process and a single result is of little clinical value. The trophoblast releases this hormone into the maternal circulation, which is metabolized and excreted by the kidneys a few days after implantation. In a properly developing pregnancy, an increase in the concentration of the β-hCG subunit, the so-called doubling time, takes place within 48 hours. In the first trimester of pregnancy, it is one of the most important indicators of proper pregnancy development. Nevertheless, you should not rely on this one parameter alone, let alone make decisions about pregnancy. There are a certain percentage of cases in which human chorionic gonadotrophin levels are abnormal in normal pregnancy. Only a comprehensive interpretation of diagnostic data allows for a good interpretation of the condition and prognosis of the developing pregnancy (Wang et al., 2020).

Many recent studies on human chorionic gonadotropin hCG prove that this hormone plays an essential role in the correct implantation of the fetus and the further development of pregnancy. It takes part in the regulation of numerous functions of various types of endometrial cells and more, and in the control of very important phenomena related to the development of pregnancy.

Moreover, it is also involved in carcinogenesis. In addition to pregnancy, it is secreted by both trophoblastic and non-trophoblastic neoplasms. The beta subunit, the secretion of which is characteristic of tumors of various origins, is of particular importance here. It is presumed that, as it is during pregnancy, hCG acts as a regulator of cell formation and apoptosis, contributing to the development of immune tolerance of the mother's organism to the fetus and tumor antigens. The mentioned angiogenic function is also reflected in the neoplastic processes. Despite these numerous negative effects of action during tumor development, hCG may show various counter-positive effects.

A thorough understanding of the function of the chorionic gonadotropin can lead to many modern medical applications of this hormone. Based on the current literature, attention should be paid to the possible therapeutic use of this hormone, for example in gynecological practice related to assisted reproductive techniques. Understanding the hCG-mediated pathways should result in the future designation of new diagnostic and therapeutic strategies for both pregnancy and neoplastic disease.

References

Gonzalez N., Tulandi T. Cesarean Scar Pregnancy: A Systematic Review. *J Minim Invasive Gynecol.* 2017 Jul-Aug;24(5):731-738.

Hendriks E., MacNaughton H., MacKenzie M. C. First Trimester Bleeding: Evaluation and Management. *Am Fam Physician.* 2019 Feb 1;99(3):166-174. PMID: 30702252.

Hendriks E., Rosenberg R., Prine L. Ectopic Pregnancy: Diagnosis and Management. *Am Fam Physician.* 2020 May 15;101(10):599-606. PMID: 32412215.

Schüler-Toprak S., Treeck O., Ortmann O. Human Chorionic Gonadotropin and Breast Cancer. *Int J Mol Sci.* 2017 Jul 21;18(7):1587.

Wang Z., Gao Y., Zhang D., Li Y., Luo L., Xu Y. Predictive value of serum β-human chorionic gonadotropin for early pregnancy outcomes. *Arch Gynecol Obstet.* 2020 Jan;301(1):295-302.

Chapter 5

Aldosterone

Tadeusz Francuz, Antoni Lalewicz,
Dorota Bartusik-Aebisher* and David Aebisher
Medical College of The University of Rzeszów, Rzeszów, Poland

Abstract

In the last two decades, significant progress has been made in understanding the new biological properties of aldosterone. Aldosterone produced not only in the adrenal glands but also in the heart and blood vessel walls. It has a negative effect on the cardiovascular system, promotes the development of fibrosis in the heart and the vascular wall, it also has a pro-arrhythmogenic effect. Based on recent studies, it can be concluded that the organ complications in primary aldosteronism are caused not only by elevated blood pressure, but also by the direct damaging effects of aldosterone on the heart and vessels. The results of a multicentre study known under the acronym RALES showed that the use of the aldosterone receptor antagonist spironolactone significantly improves the prognosis in patients with heart failure. Aldosterone, as a hormone with a significant role in the long-term regulation of intravascular volume and arterial pressure, has the ability to influence important pathophysiological processes in many disease states.

Keywords: aldosterone, heart and blood vessel walls, mineralocorticosteroid, human mononuclear leukocytes (HML)

---

* Corresponding Author's Emsil: dbartusikaebisher@ur.edu.pl.

In: The Biochemical Guide to Hormones
Editor: David Aebisher
ISBN: 979-8-88697-492-8

Aldosterone is a steroid hormone produced in the glomerular layer (beneath the capsular) of the adrenal gland. It is synthesized from cholesterol derived mainly from blood plasma. It is the strongest hormone from the mineralocorticoid group, and, moreover, due to its ability to convert into cortisol, it has poor glucocorticoid properties. Its origin in the adrenal cortex is evidenced by the structure of cyclopentanoperhydrophenanthrene consisting of 17 carbon atoms, within which there are four rings (Bothou et al., 2020).

Aldosterone stimulates the reabsorption of sodium ions in the distal and collecting tubules of the kidney and stimulates the removal of potassium, magnesium and hydrogen ions with the urine, thus regulating blood pressure and water and electrolyte balance. Aldosterone does not have a specific transport protein in plasma, but forms weakly binding to albumin. Due to this property, the described hormone is quickly cleared in the liver. The presence of high affinity receptors for aldosterone (type I receptors) has been found in the parotid glands, kidneys and large intestine. The concentration of aldosterone in the human body is regulated by the renin-angiotensin system, ACTH and the concentration of potassium or sodium in the blood plasma. The normal value of aldosterone concentration in the blood plasma is within the range of 5-20 ng/dl. Too much aldosterone in the blood (aldosteronism) is seen in high blood pressure, heart failure, cirrhosis or adrenal hyperplasia. It can also be genetically determined. In the case of aldosterone deficiency, a decrease in blood volume and a decrease in blood pressure due to the decrease in the concentration of sodium ions in the blood are observed (Bothou et al., 2020).

Aldosterone affects the water and electrolyte balance in two ways. Both modes of action have the same beginning, i.e., the hormone influences the gene transcription and translation of the messenger proteins, which in the first case affect the function of the sodium channel in the renal tubules, and in the second, they affect the functioning of the inositol triphosphate system, which is an intracellular mediator in organisms. It acts as a messenger mediating the exchange of chemical information, stimulates an increase in the concentration of Ca2 + ions in the cytosol. The action of aldosterone in the first case is long-lasting and its effects are visible only after about 2 hours, while in the second case the effect is achieved after a few minutes. The main effect that aldosterone has on the water and electrolyte balance is based on the reabsorption of Na + ions and the release of K^+ and H^+ ions into the lumen in the tubules of further nephrons, which increases the volume of circulating blood and increases blood pressure. The condition in which the concentration of aldosterone is maintained for a long time slows down the retention of sodium, while the exchange of sodium ions with hydrogen ions remains at the same level, which leads to the so-called metabolic alkalosis (Hellman et al., 2019).

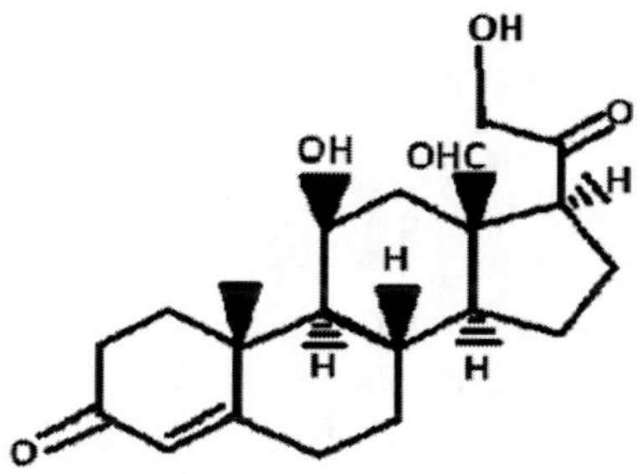

Figure 1. Chemical formula of Aldosterone.

The molecular mechanism of action of aldosterone is based on the interaction of this hormone with specific intracellular receptors for mineralocorticosteroids. Recent studies have shown a greater affinity of cortisol to the same receptors, meaning that cortisol must be inactivated before these receptors interact with aldosterone. The MR (mineralocorticosteroid) receptor contains two domains in the terminal amino acid chain: 1) the ligand binding domain, i.e., aldosterone, and 2) the DNA binding domain. After ligand is attached, the receptor-aldosterone complex is activated and migrates to the nucleus where it interacts with specific DNA sequences. The effect of this interaction is the stimulation of mRNA synthesis, which codes for so-called aldosterone-induced proteins, involved in the control of sodium transport and intracellular pH. It is a multi-stage process that requires modification of transcription, translation and protein biosynthesis. A characteristic feature of this process is the delayed action, since the effect is only observed after about 4 hours (Lim et al., 2020). In the late 1990s, the rapid (1-2 min) effect of aldosterone was described. It consists in the stimulation of sodium transport (activation of Na^+ / / H^+ antiports), an increase in the intracellular concentration of calcium ions, which leads to an increase in the cell volume and indirectly to the activation of protein kinase C. This phenomenon has been demonstrated on the model of human mononuclear leukocytes (HML), endothelial cells and vascular smooth muscle cells. The mechanism of this action is different from that described previously and does not involve interaction with the cell genome (Schilbach et al., 2019).

Rapid stimulation of sodium transport occurs through direct interaction with other types of receptors located in the cytoplasmic membrane. The presence of such receptors has been demonstrated in the preparations of HML membranes and vascular smooth muscle cells, as well as in renal cells. The binding characteristics and high selectivity (1000–10,000 times greater affinity for aldosterone compared to the glucocorticosteroids cortisol and corticosterone) suggest that it is a different type of receptor, different from intracellular MR receptors.

The rapid effect of aldosterone is associated with a marked stimulation of protein kinase C and an increase in the concentration of inositol 1,4,5-triphosphate, which is already observed after 30-60 sec. from aldosterone application. The consequence of this phenomenon is a significant increase in the concentration of calcium ions, released from the endoplasmic reticulum pool and partially transported from the extracellular space. The inhibition of this phenomenon by neomycin, which is an inhibitor of phospholipase C, also indicates the participation of this enzyme in the intracellular signaling cascade. A mechanism is also suggested, at the present hypothetical stage, in which a specific G protein and protein tyrosine kinase are involved. A quick effect, bypassing the mechanism of interaction with the genetic material, is already observed at very low concentrations of aldosterone (Seccia et al., 2019).

In the last two decades, significant progress has been made in understanding the new biological properties of aldosterone. Aldosterone has been shown to be produced not only in the adrenal glands but also in the heart and blood vessel walls. It has a negative effect on the cardiovascular system, promotes the development of fibrosis in the heart and the vascular wall, it also has a pro-arrhythmogenic effect. In recent years, the relationship of aldosterone with the development of primary arterial hypertension and primary hyperaldosteronism has been emphasized, and research into its participation in the course of heart failure or heart attack is also being developed. The role of aldosterone in the pathophysiology of primary hypertension is postulated. Recently, it has been accepted that the pathogenesis of essential hypertension is complex and multifactorial.

The demonstration of new properties of the discussed hormone suggests that it may play a role as a pathogenetic factor, especially in the development of organ complications of primary hypertension. Primary aldosteronism is a form of arterial hypertension that allows the direct effect of aldosterone on the cardiovascular system to be traced. Patients with excessive, autonomic secretion of aldosterone in the course of adenoma or adrenal hyperplasia are often characterized by severe, refractory arterial hypertension.

Based on recent studies, it can be concluded that the organ complications in primary aldosteronism are caused not only by elevated blood pressure, but also by the direct damaging effects of aldosterone on the heart and vessels. It has long been known that in the course of heart failure, aldosterone secretion is increased, which contributes to the increased reabsorption of sodium and water in the kidneys and leads to an increase in volemia. The results of a multicentre study known under the acronym RALES showed that the use of the aldosterone receptor antagonist spironolactone significantly improves the prognosis in patients with heart failure.

It has also been shown that the new aldosterone antagonist eplerenone has a positive effect on the prognosis of patients with left ventricular dysfunction after a myocardial infarction. In summary, aldosterone, as a hormone with a significant role in the long-term regulation of intravascular volume and arterial pressure, has the ability to influence important pathophysiological processes in many disease states.

References

Bothou C., Beuschlein F., Spyroglou A. Links between aldosterone excess and metabolic complications: A comprehensive review. *Diabetes Metab.* 2020 Feb;46(1):1-7.

Hellman P., Björklund P., Åkerström T. Aldosterone-Producing Adenomas. *Vitam Horm.* 2019;109:407-431.

Lim J. S., Rainey W. E. The Potential Role of Aldosterone-Producing Cell Clusters in Adrenal Disease. *Horm Metab Res.* 2020 Jun;52(6):427-434.

Schilbach K., Junnila R. K., Bidlingmaier M. Aldosterone to Renin Ratio as Screening Tool in Primary Aldosteronism. *Exp Clin Endocrinol Diabetes.* 2019 Feb;127(2-03):84-92.

Seccia T. M., Caroccia B., Maiolino G., Cesari M., Rossi G. P. Arterial Hypertension, Aldosterone, and Atrial Fibrillation. *Curr Hypertens Rep.* 2019 Nov 18;21(12):94.

Chapter 6

Corticosteroids

**Sara Bień, Dorota Bartusik-Aebisher*
and David Aebisher**
Medical College of The University of Rzeszów, Poland

Abstract

Corticosteroids are steroid hormones produced in the banded and reticular layers of the adrenal cortex under the influence of the pituitary hormone adrenocorticotropin (ACTH). During stress, there is an increased secretion of ACTH, and thus glucorticoids. Glucocorticoids cannot remain elevated for long periods. This condition can lead to Cushing's syndrome. The excess of the hormone also leads to bone autolysis, which leads to osteoporosis and accelerates the basic rhythm recorded during electroencephalography, causes mental disorders. Glucocorticoids are used in diseases where the anti-inflammatory effect is beneficial and the immune system is weakened. The action of corticosteroids is extensive, they affect the tissues and therefore the functioning of the organs and systems of the body. Corticosteroids are recommended by doctors to treat conditions such as Addison's disease with adrenal insufficiency. Although corticosteroids are hormones necessary for the proper functioning of the body and are used as therapeutic agents in many diseases, it should be remembered that their use may be associated with a number of side effects.

Keywords: adrenocorticotropin, corticosteroids, Cushing's syndrome, steroid, glucocorticosteroids

---

* Corresponding Author's Email: dbartusikaebisher@ur.edu.pl.

In: The Biochemical Guide to Hormones
Editor: David Aebisher
ISBN: 979-8-88697-492-8

Corticosteroids (corticosteroids, glucorticoids, corticosteroids, corticosteroids) are steroid hormones produced in the banded and reticular layers of the adrenal cortex under the influence of the pituitary hormone adrenocorticotropin (ACTH). They include: cortisol, corticosterone, and cortisone (Figure 1). They exhibit strong and diverse activities, they are responsible for the transformation of proteins, carbohydrates and fats, with their help they are treated all kinds of diseases. As drugs, they have anti-inflammatory, antiallergic and immunosuppressive effects, and also correspond to the hormones of the adrenal glands that are produced by the human body. Over secretion of corticosteroids causes hypercortisolemia, a disease called Cushing's syndrome, while insufficiency causes Addison's disease. Glucorticoids increase protein catabolism, hepatic glycogenesis, gluconeogenesis, glucose-6-phosphatase activity and blood glucose levels. They can aggravate the symptoms of diabetes by exerting an anti-insulin effect in peripheral tissues, increase the content of plasma lipids and increase the formation of ketone bodies. This effect does not occur in healthy subjects as it is suppressed by the normal secretion of insulin. Corticosteroids reduce the absorption of calcium from the gut and increase its excretion in the urine, which can cause bone disorders such as osteoporosis. In higher concentrations, they cause a minerralocorticoid effect such as sodium retention in the body, as well as edema. Corticosteroids have a permissive effect, i.e., even a small amount of them is necessary for the occurrence of many metabolic reactions, even though they are not directly involved in them (Bleecker et al., 2020).

- they inhibit the secretion of adrenocorticotropin, and the secretion of corticosteroids depends on ACTH. Secretion of the adrenal cortex can be stimulated by angiotensin II, including the secretion of aldosterone. Serotonin, vasopressin and VIP also have a stimulating effect, but have no effect on corticosteroids,
- they reactivate blood vessels that can become permeable to colloids at the moment of expanding. This happens when adrenal insufficiency occurs and the smooth muscle layer of blood vessels becomes insensitive to adrenaline and noradrenaline released from noradrenergic endings,
- they also reverse changes in the nervous system that result from adrenal insufficiency,
- they reduce the number of eosinophils in the blood by increasing their uptake and storage in the spleen and also in the lungs. They also

reduce the number of basophils and increase neutrophils, erythrocyte platelets. They reduce the number of lymphocytes and the size of the thymus and lymph nodes,

- they operate when there is a risk of water poisoning in the organism. This is because it is difficult to excrete excess water in the presence of adrenal insufficiency. If the patient is not given glucocorticoids in time, he develops a high fever due to glucose infusion, which may be fatal.
- they inhibit the inflammatory reaction after tissue damage and the symptoms of allergy that occurs with the release of histamine. They can be used topically by injection into an inflamed joint,
- high doses reduce the secretion of growth hormone and TSH,
- in utero they accelerate the production of surfactant in the lungs (Goldman et al., 2020).

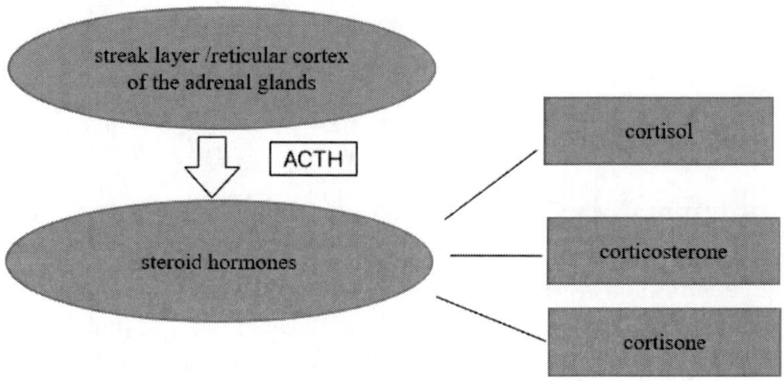

Figure 1. Steroid hormones produced in the banded and reticular layers of the adrenal cortex under the influence of ACTH. They include: cortisol, corticosterone, and cortisone. [Own study].

As mentioned above, corticosteroids inhibit the secretion of ACTH, and the secretion of glucorticosteroids depends on adencorticotropin. During stress, there is an increased secretion of ACTH, and thus glucorticoids. This may be because stressors activate the sympathetic nervous system and corticosteroids will be necessary to maintain the responsiveness of the muscle membrane. They will also determine the full activity of catecholamines in the mobilization of free fatty acids, which are a source of energy. Glucocorticoids cannot remain elevated for long periods. This condition can lead to Cushing's syndrome. The disease may be ACTH dependent and independent of the disease. The independent form may be caused by the presence of adrenal tumors or by their hypertrophy. The dependent form will be caused by the tumor of the anterior pituitary gland, which is responsible for the secretion of ACTH. Other tumors, such as the lung, may also be the cause. Excessive corticosteroids may have a mineralocorticoid effect. If the cause of the disease is ACTH hypersecretion, the secretion of deoxycorticosterone will also be increased. Retained water, salt and fat build-up will result in a distinctive facial appearance known as the full moon. The excess of the hormone also leads to bone autolysis, which leads to osteoporosis and accelerates the basic rhythm recorded during electroencephalography, causes mental disorders (Rice et al., 2017).

Substitution Therapy

Corticosteroid drugs are administered in the presence of adrenal hormone deficiencies. To mimic the natural secretion even better, mineralocorticosteroids and androgens are also often administered.

Anti-Inflammatory Drugs

Glucocorticoids are used in diseases where the anti-inflammatory effect is beneficial and the immune system is weakened. Examples in which corticosteroids are worth using are: proliferative diseases, local inflammations related to dermatological problems, counteracting transplant rejection, autoimmune diseases, anaphylactic shock, bronchial asthma, congenital adrenal hyperplasia, neoplastic diseases. Corticosteroids in the human body are exclusively produced in the adrenal cortex, a structure weighing up to 4 grams. Glucocorticosteroids are produced in the banded layer and in a small portion of the reticular layer. The main corticosteroid hormones are cortisol and corticosterone. If the adrenal cortex was reduced, a person would be at risk of dying in 3-14 days (van Paassen et al., 2020).

In laboratories, glucocorticosteroids are synthesized with an activity 30 times stronger than their natural ones, including dexamethasone, prednisone, and methylprednisone. The action of corticosteroids is extensive, they affect the tissues and therefore the functioning of the organs and systems of the body. The most important roles are primarily controlling the metabolic conversion of carbohydrates, proteins and fats, reducing inflammatory processes in the body, increasing the activity of liver enzymes causing the breakdown of glycogen to maintain the proper level and controlling the functions of the circulatory system, the central nervous system and the immune system. Corticosteroids are recommended by doctors to treat conditions such as Addison's disease with adrenal insufficiency, urticaria, asthma, insect venom allergies, gastrointestinal diseases such as celiac disease and inflammatory nephritis. We also use them in hematological diseases: leukemia, lymphomas, rheumatology and skin diseases, e.g., atopic inflammation. Although corticosteroids are hormones necessary for the proper functioning of the body and are used as therapeutic agents in many diseases, it should be remembered that their use may be associated with a number of side effects (Yang et al., 2020).

References

Bleecker E R, Menzies-Gow A N, Price D B, Bourdin A, Sweet S, Martin A L, Alacqua M, Tran T N. Systematic Literature Review of Systemic Corticosteroid Use for Asthma Management. *Am. J. Respir. Crit. Care Med.* 2020 Feb 1;201(3):276-293.

Goldman C, Judson M A. Corticosteroid refractory sarcoidosis. *Respir. Med.* 2020 Sep;171:106081.

Rice J B, White A G, Scarpati L M, Wan G, Nelson WW. Long-term Systemic Corticosteroid Exposure: A Systematic Literature Review. *Clin. Ther.* 2017 Nov;39 (11):2216-2229.

van Paassen J, Vos J S, Hoekstra E M, Neumann K M I, Boot P C, Arbous S M. Corticosteroid use in COVID-19 patients: a systematic review and meta-analysis on clinical outcomes. *Crit. Care.* 2020 Dec 14;24(1):696.

Yang J W, Yang L, Luo R G, Xu J F. Corticosteroid administration for viral pneumonia: COVID-19 and beyond. *Clin. Microbiol. Infect.* 2020 Sep;26(9):1171-1177.

Chapter 7

Antidiuretic Hormone (Vasopressin)

Aleksandra Faff, Dorota Bartusik-Aebisher*
and David Aebisher
Medical College of The University of Rzeszów, Poland

Abstract

Vasopressin is an antidiuretic hormone that actively participates in blood pressure regulation, concentrates urine due to water reabsorption by stimulation of receptors. A disturbed amount of vasopressin may lead to complications related to its deficiency or excess. Too much of this hormone manifests itself in Schwartz-Bartter syndrome. Antidiuretic hormone is also used in the case of vasoplegic shock, because strong vasopressor activity is associated with the activation of V1 receptors. One of the diseases caused by ADH deficiency, i.e., nephrogenic diabetes insipidus, is caused by a defect of vasopressin V2 receptors, which are insensitive to its proper secretion and there are no specific actions in the body that are responsible. Vasopressin analogues or antagonists are often used in the treatment of such disorders.

Keywords: vasopressin, antidiuretic hormone, receptors, kidney, catecholamines

Vasopressin is an antidiuretic hormone that is a cyclic nonapeptide made of nine amino acid residues. It is produced by the hypothalamic and paraventricular nuclei, it is stored in the posterior pituitary gland and from

* Corresponding Author's Email: dbartusikaebisher@ur.edu.pl.

In: The Biochemical Guide to Hormones
Editor: David Aebisher
ISBN: 979-8-88697-492-8

there it is also released into the circulatory system. The stimuli that stimulate its release are the increase in blood plasma and cerebrospinal fluid osmolality, hypovolemia, drop in blood pressure, decrease in circulating blood volume and the stimulation of ADH-producing neurons by angiotensin II (Bankir et al., 2017). Vasopressin actively participates in blood pressure regulation, concentrates urine due to water reabsorption by stimulation of V2 receptors (wall of distal tubules and collecting tubules) [Figure 1]. and V1 (vessel wall). Its function is also to change the activity of hepatic glycogenolysis, central regulation of food intake and participation in the regulation of insulin and glucagon secretion (Bankir et al., 2017). The antidiuretic hormone also

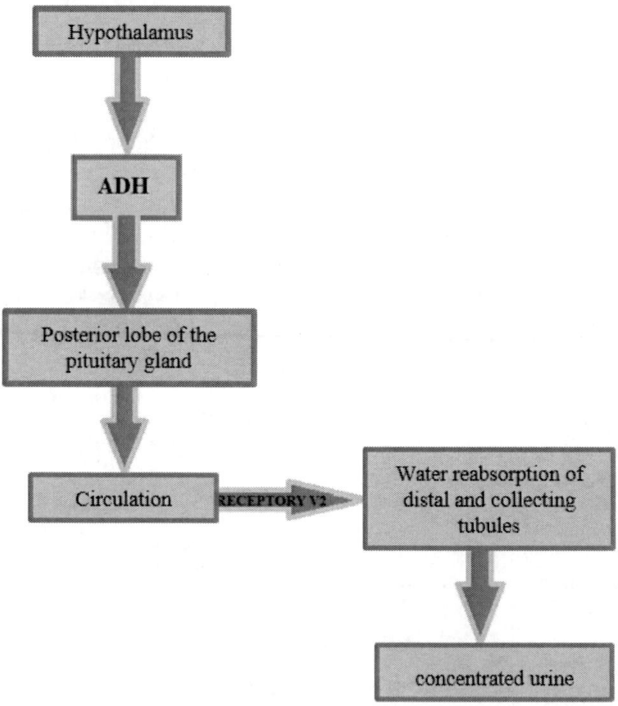

Figure 1. Urine concentrating process under the influence of vasopressin produced by the hypothalamus and secreted by the posterior lobe of the pituitary gland. [Own elaboration].

stimulates the release of atrial natriuretic factor through the action of V1, while atrial natriuretic factor reduces the release of vasopressin and inhibits the antidiuretic effect of vasopressin, which maintains the tonicity of the extracellular fluid and acts as a feedback loop. A disturbed amount of vasopressin may lead to complications related to its deficiency or excess (Christ-Crain et al., 2019). Deficiency or lack of adiuretin causes dia-central diabetes insipidus when it concerns errors at the level of the hypothalamus / pituitary gland and kidney, and the insensitivity (resistance) of the renal tubules to the action of this hormone. However, too much of this hormone manifests itself in Schwartz-Bartter syndrome (Christ-Crain et al., 2019).

The release of vasopressin stimulates many stimuli. The first is the change in serum osmolality. There are special nerve cells in the hypothalamus, osmoreceptors, which are highly sensitive to these changes (Li et al., 2019). They are associated with nerve cells that secrete and produce vasopressin. Already a 1 percent change in osmolality causes a change in the amount of antidiuretic hormone secreted. Normal serum osmolality in healthy individuals ranges from approximately 285 to 300 milliosmoles per kilogram (mOsm / kg). As a result of an increase in serum osmolality, for example due to dehydration due to excessive sweating, diarrhea, vomiting or prolonged and intense physical exertion, osmoreceptors are stimulated, which leads to the separation of vasopressin from molecules of neurophysin, with which ADH is loosely bound in secretory cells. The next stage is the release of this hormone from the posterior pituitary gland, which results in increased water reabsorption in the renal tubules (Li et al., 2019). The opposite effect is caused by a decrease in serum osmolality, which is often caused by excessive hydration or diseases such as diabetes. This leads to an inhibition of the osmoreceptors, a reduction in vasopressin secretion and an increase in water excretion. The thirst center, with which the osmoreceptors are also associated, is governed by the alteration of the serum osmolality in the same way as the antidiuretic hormone (Ukor et al., 2019). The release of vasopressin also occurs as a result of a change in blood volume, specifically a decrease in blood volume. In the carotid sinus, which is associated with each carotid artery located in the upper part of the neck, and in a group of specialized cells in the left atrium of the heart, there are pressure sensors or baroreceptors. Their stimulation occurs when the blood volume increases, leading to stretching of the tissues of the carotid sinus and the left atrium. The nerves in the baroreceptors transmit impulses to the nerve cells in the testes where vasopressin is produced and its secretion is reduced, resulting in an increased amount of water. The opposite effect is a reduced amount of excreted water due to increased water reabsorption in the renal tubules, which is due to the increased secretion of vasopressin. This is due to a reduction in blood volume, the carotid sinus, and the left atrium (Ukor et al., 2019). This enables the blood volume to be equalized. Stimuli that also influence ADH secretion are certain drugs, such as opiate drugs, as well as pain and increased stress. It is also released in response to shock states, but its relative deficiency is found in situations of prolonged shock which dilates the blood vessels, for example in severe sepsis. In such a situation, the use of exogenous vasopressin causes a vasopressin effect, even in the case of doses that do not affect the blood pressure value in healthy people. This enables the use of ADH in the treatment of septic shock. Antidiuretic hormone is also used in the case of vasoplegic shock, because strong vasopressor activity is associated with the activation of V1 receptors. They are located in the smooth muscles of the vessels. Vasopressin has a very similar effect to catecholamines, because it can also inhibit pathological processes occurring in states of shock, i.e., vasodilation. The interest in its therapeutic effect in treating tremors due to ventricular fibrillation, hypovolemia and sepsis is constantly growing. Vasopressin is also an essential hormone that is involved in the maintenance of cardiovascular homeostasis. It is used therapeutically, mainly due to its antidiuretic properties and vasoconstrictive effects. A synthetic analogue of vasopressin is desmopressin, which has a stronger antidiuretic effect and a lower vasoconstrictor effect than ADH (Zeynalov et al., 2020).

The release of vasopressin is regulated by three V-receptor subtypes, which are isoforms. We distinguish between V1a, V1b and V2. Each of them has a specific function in the action of the antidiuretic hormone. V1a receptor activation triggers vasoconstriction and is also responsible for inhibiting renal sodium reabsorption and inducing natriuresis. Stimulation of the V1b receptor induces the secretion of potassium in the distal sections of the distal sections and in the initial sections of the collecting ducts, and has an effect on behavior and modulation of mood. In turn, the activated V2 receptor is involved in the regulation of the osmotic concentration of urine, as it increases the osmotic permeability in the collecting duct, which passes through the epithelial cells and stimulates sodium reabsorption in the leg of the ascending loop of Henle. In the event of stress or disease, among others, excessive secretion of vasopressin may occur, which often triggers harmful pathways that can lead to hyponatremia and emerging cerebral edema, especially in the case of pathological conditions such as subarachnoid hemorrhage, stroke or liver disease. In such situations, the action of V1a and V2 receptors may be enhanced (Zeynalov et al., 2020).

One of the diseases caused by ADH deficiency, i.e., nephrogenic diabetes insipidus, is caused by a defect of vasopressin V2 receptors, which are insensitive to its proper secretion and there are no specific actions in the body that are responsible. Vasopressin analogues or antagonists are often used in the treatment of such disorders.

References

Bankir L, Bichet D G, Morgenthaler N G. Vasopressin: physiology, assessment and osmosensation. *J. Intern. Med.* 2017 Oct;282(4):284-297.

Christ-Crain M. Vasopressin and Copeptin in health and disease. *Rev. Endocr. Metab. Disord.* 2019 Sep;20(3):283-294.

Li D T, Habtemichael E N, Bogan J S. Vasopressin inactivation: Role of insulin- regulated aminopeptidase. *Vitam. Horm.* 2020;113:101-128.

Ukor I F, Walley K R. Vasopressin in Vasodilatory Shock. *Crit. Care Clin.* 2019 Apr;35(2):247-261.

Zeynalov E, Jones S M, Elliott J P. Vasopressin and vasopressin receptors in brain edema. *Vitam. Horm.* 2020;113:291-312.

Chapter 8

Adrenocorticotropic Hormone (ACTH)

Aleksandra Flak, Dorota Bartusik-Aebisher[*]
and David Aebisher
Medical College of The University of Rzeszów, Poland

Abstract

Adrenocorticotropin is a hormone secreted from the anterior pituitary gland under the influence of the hypothalamic hormone corticoliberin. ACTH hormone is necessary for the proper functioning of our body, because it affects its many aspects as well as the functioning of other organs. Most ACTH-secreting pituitary tumors are microadenomas, half of them below 5 mm in diameter, and their MRI detectability ranges from 35-60%. T". Additionally, ACTH inhibits cell proliferation and, as the research shows, it has anti-inflammatory and anti-allergic properties. Also, it is often used in the treatment of Addison's disease, i.e., adrenal insufficiency. However, the choice of ACTH therapy may cause various side reactions, such as: edema due to mineral disturbances, circulatory disorders, allergies, increased blood pressure and a decrease in gastric pH. It should be remembered that for the correct interpretation of the results, the serum cortisol level should be measured together with the ACTH level test. Then the comparison of these two values allows to realistically and correctly determine the cause of the disorders.

Keywords: hormone, adrenocorticotropin, adrenocorticotropic hormone (ACTH), proopiomelanocortin

---

[*] Corresponding Author's Email: dbartusikaebisher@ur.edu.pl.

In: The Biochemical Guide to Hormones
Editor: David Aebisher
ISBN: 979-8-88697-492-8

ACTH is an adrenocorticotropin. It is a peptide hormone that comes from proopiomelanocortin – POMc for short and is also classified as melanocortin, in addition, ACTH is converted intracellularly into a stimulating hormone. Adrenocorticotropin is a hormone secreted from the anterior pituitary gland under the influence of the hypothalamic hormone corticoliberin. Adrenocorticotropin works to stimulate the production of cortisol by the adrenal glands (specifically the cortex of the adrenal glands), and ACTH is also produced by other cells, such as macrophages (Crane et al., 2020).

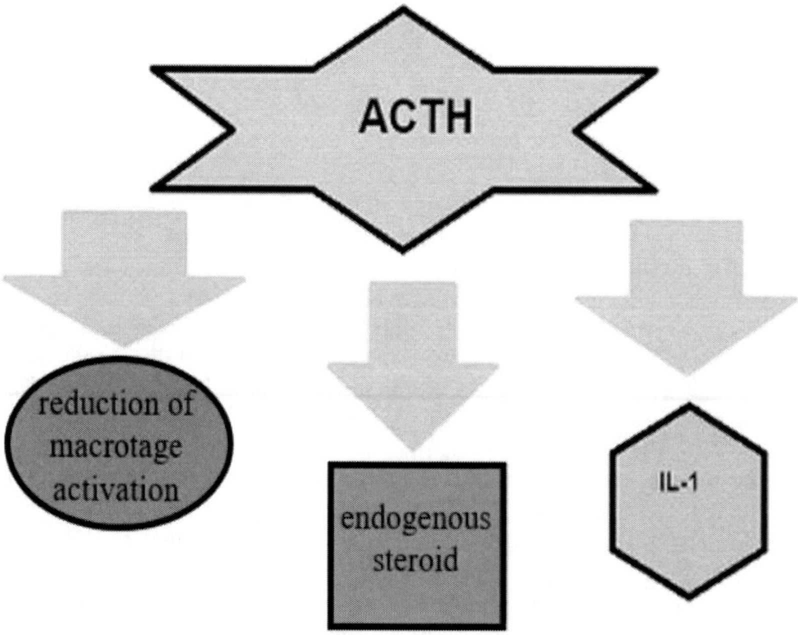

Figure 1. ACTH operation. [Own elaboration].

The hormone is made up of approximately 39 amino acids. ACTH works by negative feedback through endogenous opioids. An important aspect of this hormone is its circadian rhythm of secretion, which is sometimes disturbed, for example, by stress or anxiety (Crane et al., 2020). The concentration of ACTH in the blood is used in the diagnosis of diseases of the adrenal glands. The reason for the low concentration of this hormone may be adrenal damage – secondary insufficiency, and high levels of ectopic ACTH production or excessive production by the pituitary gland (Daoussis et al., 2020).

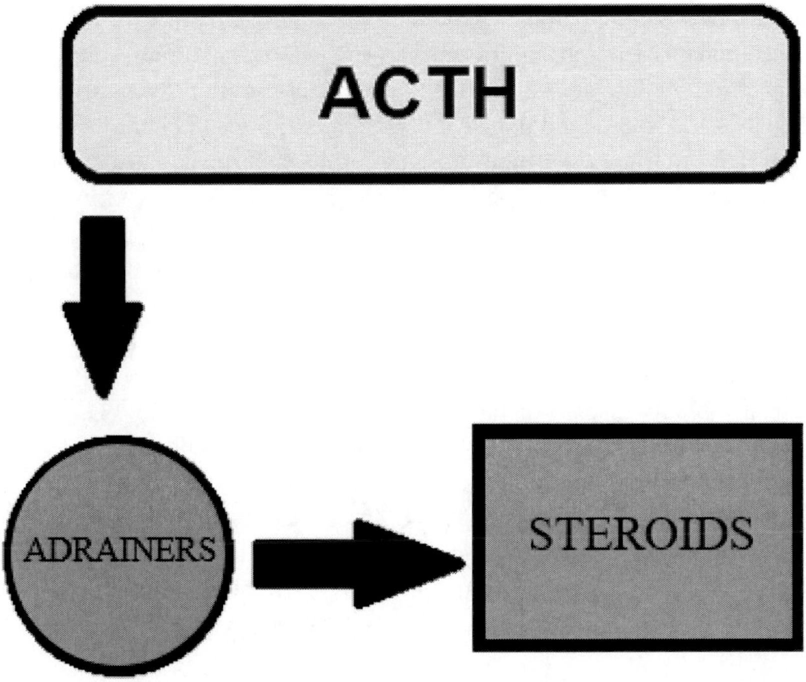

Figure 2. Effect of ACTH on the adrenal glands. [Own study].

In states of excessive ACTH secretion, excessive pigmentation of the skin appears, which is the reason for the action of this hormone on skin melanocytes, it is related to the fact that adrenocorticotropin contains MSH sequences. Abnormalities related to the level of ACTH concentration and level can also cause: adrenal tumor that autonomously secretes cortisol, pituitary tumor that autonomously secretes ACTH, Addison's disease, Cushing's syndrome. However, the most visible changes in ACTH concentration occur in an intense stressful situation, which is why ACTH is sometimes called a stress hormone (Daoussis et al., 2020).

ACTH has a neural mechanism of effectiveness mainly in the clinic. This mechanism is independent of the steroidal effects of neurological disorders such as, for example, infantile contractions, myoclonic seizures in infants. ACTH is a neurotransmitter, growth factor, and also a neuromodulator. ACTH has an extremely interesting and important function in our body, such as: ACTH in combination with receptors in the brain affects their metabolism, moreover, ACTH influences the growth of cultured neurons. ACTH has neurochemical properties that can alter neurotransmission, as well as anticonvulsant, antmyoclonic, and neurophysiological properties. There is currently evidence based on effects on the CNS and the presence of ACTH neuropeptide binding sites in the CNS. Low concentrations of these peptides in the CNS and CNS receptors have very high affinity and very low capacity. This greatly interferes with the presentation of such receptor sites at direct binding sites with the use of peptides. The action of a peptide hormone such as adrenocorticotropin, ACTH for short in stimulating the production of glucocorticoids by the adrenal glands, is a very important physiological process, but depends on the genetic component – the ACTH receptor or the melanocortin 2 receptor. Genetic abnormalities that cause errors in this receptor or protein which is necessary for its expression on the cell surface lead to the deadly disease of familial glucocorticoid deficiency (Daoussis et al., 2020). Overexpression of this receptor or the inability to desensitize it is observed in adrenal adenomas, as well as in hypertrophy associated with the overproduction of glucocorticoids, the so-called Cushing's syndrome. The disorders shown are extremely rare, however, there is a lot of evidence that the hypothalamic-pituitary-adrenal axis is overactive or in some circumstances completely inactive in situations such as depression or septic shock (D'Alonzo et al., 2018).

The cause of these disorders is complex and multifactorial, but there is substantial evidence that the basis of this phenomenon is an altered ACTH receptor response to ACTH. Understanding the basics of the response to ACTH may contribute to a better understanding of these types of disorders and possibly enable hypothalamic-pituitary-adrenal control in such situations. There is a theory that blocking the ACTH receptor by a blocking antibody or drug will result in cortical adrenalectomy with a relative reduction in mineralocorticoid hormone production. You would experience symptoms similar to a familial type 1 glucocorticoid deficiency, an autosomal recessive disease caused by mutations that inactivate the adrenal receptor for ACTH, known as the melanocortin 2 receptor (MC2R). In addition, there is also a theory that blocking MC2R may allow much lower doses of glucocorticoids to be used in the treatment of congenital adrenal hyperplasia, abbreviated as CAH, due to hydroxylase deficiency, which will result in better adult growth than blocking the ACTH receptor may also be used in the treatment of the syndrome (D'Alonzo et al., 2018). Cushing as a result of excessive pituitary and ectopic ACTH production. A lot of experiments that are related to ACTH-related peptides and including tests show that ACTH-related peptides have a neuroactive effect on activities such as learning, motivation, and better concentration. Additionally, the ACTH neuropeptide influences social behavior and has antiepileptic properties by binding to opiates. Other effects on the central nervous system that can be seen after intracranial administration include grooming, stretching, yawning and sexual behavior. The effects mainly relate to the N-terminal part of ACTH which is separate from the peripheral corticotropic effect. Several substitutions in the ACTH- (4-9) sequence have resulted in a loss of endocrine effects. ACTH peptide also has a neurotrophic effect, which makes it affect the regeneration of damaged nerve cells. Animal studies have shown a beneficial effect of semi-chronic treatment with ACTH analogue on regeneration of damaged nerves in animals. This effect is found in the ACTH- (6-10) sequence. The neurotrophic effect is visible both at the level of sensory and motor functions, and this effect is also present in other neuropathies as a result of e.g., diabetes or chemotherapy (Fukuoka et al., 2020).

To sum up, ACTH, the hormone called adrenocorticotropin, is essential for the proper functioning of the body. ACTH4-10 is much better in protecting podocytes from damage caused by ADR by increasing the secretion of IL-10. moreover, "15% of patients with ectopic ACTH secretion have abnormalities in the pituitary gland on MRI. Most ACTH-secreting pituitary tumors are microadenomas, half of them below 5 mm in diameter, and their MRI detectability ranges from 35-60%. T "Additionally, ACTH inhibits cell proliferation and, as the research shows, it has anti-inflammatory and anti-allergic properties. In addition, it is often used, among others in the treatment of Addison's disease, i.e., adrenal insufficiency. However, the choice of ACTH therapy may cause various side reactions, such as: edema due to mineral disturbances, circulatory disorders, allergies, increased blood pressure and a decrease in gastric pH (Ohara et al., 2020). It should be remembered that for the correct interpretation of the results, the serum cortisol level should be measured together with the ACTH level test. Then the comparison of these two values allows to realistically and correctly determine the cause of the disorders. Another important aspect is the correct interpretation of the test results. For example, in a person with symptoms of hyperadrenocorticism along with a high concentration of cortisol in the serum, the ACTH level is reduced, this is due to the fact that it is primary adrenal hyperfunction, while if the ACTH level is high, the cause is secondary adrenal hyperfunction (Ohara et al., 2020).

References

Crane A B, Sharon Y, Chu D S. Use of Adrenocorticotropic Hormone in Ophthalmology. *J. Ocul. Pharmacol. Ther.* 2020 Nov;36(9):661-667.

D'Alonzo R, Rigante D, Mencaroni E, Esposito S. West Syndrome: A Review and Guide for Paediatricians. *Clin. Drug. Investig.* 2018 Feb;38(2):113-124.

Daoussis D, Bogdanos D P, Dimitroulas T, Sakkas L, Andonopoulos AP. Adrenocorticotropic hormone: an effective "natural" biologic therapy for acute gout? *Rheumatol. Int.* 2020 Dec;40(12):1941-1947.

Fukuoka H, Shichi H, Yamamoto M, Takahashi Y. The Mechanisms Underlying Autonomous Adrenocorticotropic Hormone Secretion in Cushing's Disease. *Int. J. Mol. Sci.* 2020 Nov 30;21(23):9132.

Ohara N, Kobayashi M, Tuchida M, Koda R, Yoneoka Y, Iino N. Isolated Adrenocorticotropic Hormone Deficiency and Primary Hypothyroidism in a Patient Undergoing Long-Term Hemodialysis: A Case Report and Literature Review. *Am. J. Case Rep.* 2020 Apr 28;21:e922376.

Chapter 9

Growth Hormone (GH)

Julia Florek, Dorota Bartusik-Aebisher*
and David Aebisher
Medical College of The University of Rzeszów, Poland

Abstract

Growth hormone enhances the growth of long bones and organs. It also stimulates glycogenolysis and glucose secretion from the liver and positive effect on the condition of the skin, concentration and mood. Growth hormone is the most important factor in regulating weight gain in the body. Its deficiency leads to the development of severely disabling dysfunctions, such as dwarfism, while its too high concentration may lead to acromegaly or gigantism. The norms of growth hormone levels differ for adults and children: they range from about 1 to 12 ng / ml for adults and from about 10 to 30 ng / ml for children. GH used for a long time may lead to hypoglycaemia and an increase in the concentration of free fatty acids in the plasma, and in extreme cases even to the development of acromegaly. Taking supplements containing the so-called growth hormone precursors and an appropriate diet that increases the synthesis of somatropin in the body.

Keywords: hormone, growth hormone (GH), somatropin, growth hormone inhibiting hormone (GHIH), somatomedins, hypoglycaemia

---

* Corresponding Author's Email: dbartusikaebisher@ur.edu.pl.

In: The Biochemical Guide to Hormones
Editor: David Aebisher
ISBN: 979-8-88697-492-8

It is a substance that stimulates the synthesis of nucleic acids, thus enhancing DNA replication and mitotic processes. It enhances the growth of long bones and organs. It also stimulates glycogenolysis and glucose secretion from the liver, and the production of liver-mediating proteins – somatomedins – otherwise known as insulin-like growth factors (IGF-1, IGF-2), which indirectly influences the lipolysis process in adipose tissues). Therefore, it causes an increase in the secretion of insulin by the pancreas. In addition, it has a positive effect on the condition of the skin, concentration and mood. Its production depends on age, sex, glandular pituitary function, and even the time of day, because it is produced most intensively at night, during deep sleep (Aguiar-Oliveira et al., 2019).

In terms of structure, GH belongs to the polypeptide hormones. It consists of 191 amino acid residues and has two disulfide bridges in its structure. It has a molecular weight of 21.5 kDa and a quad helix structure. Human growth hormone differs from its counterparts in other species. It is produced by eosinophilic cells (Mallory staining) of the anterior pituitary gland. Its production is regulated by liberins and statins in the hypothalamus. Somatoliberin – stimulates eosinophilic cells to produce it, while somatostatin – inhibits it (Caicedo et al., 2018).

Somatropin is the primary hormonal (non-genetic) growth factor in the body. The structure of its molecule and the scope of its action are very similar to prolactin and placental lactogen (hPL – human placental latogen). It is also worth adding that it shows species specificity, which means that the obtained hormone from different species of mammals will show a different biological activity, immunological properties, and a different biochemical structure. The only example of having a similar structure of active centers, and thus a similar effect of growth hormones obtained from individuals of different species, are human and monkey hormones (human GH stimulates the growth of a monkey and vice versa). This similarity is probably related to the specificity of somatropin receptors in primates (Martínez-Moreno et al., 2020).

The concentration of hormones in human serum often depends on age, sex and circadian rhythm, it is no different in this case. The highest concentration is reached in the womb and in newborns, but it decreases after the end of puberty (however, it is still higher than in adults). In the case of gender differences – in women (especially before ovulation), it reaches a higher concentration, which is related to the stimulating effect of estradiol. GH secretion peaks at night, in NREM slow-wave sleep, but drops during the day. The secretion of growth hormone is regulated by the hypothalamus hormones, which have the opposite effect: growth hormone relasing hormone (GHRH) and growth hormone inhibiting hormone, also known as somatostatin (GHIH – growth hormone inhibiting hormone). There is a negative feedback loop between the above-mentioned and GH. In addition to the hypothalamic-pituitary mechanism, there are many factors regulating the secretion of somatropin, the stimulants include: decrease in glucose concentration and FFA concentration (free fatty acids), increase in serum amino acids, hunger, ghrelin, exercise, stress, estrogens , androgens, dopamine, acetylcholine, serotonin, enkephalins, alpha-adrenergic agonists, while the inhibitory effect is shown by: an increase in serum glucose and FFA, somatomedin, GH, cortisol, beta-adrenergic agonists (Martínez-Moreno et al., 2020).

The main target of GH action is the liver, which in response releases somatomedins such as IGF-1 and IGF-2. It also acts directly on muscles and connective adipose tissue. The effect of the hormone's action on the membrane receptors of the above-mentioned organs is the activation of the intracellular cascade of the JAK2-STAT pathway. The components of this pathway are activated by somatotropin-dependent cytoplasmic kinases and become active transcription factors that reach the cell nucleus and activate genes responsible for the biological effects of growth hormone. Due to the action of enhancing the synthesis of appropriate mRNA, and later proteins and enzymes, the effects of this hormone are visible only after a few hours or days (Ranke et al., 2018). GH, as previously mentioned, is the main and the most important factor in the human body, which stimulates weight gain, tissues: nervous, lymph, and the growth of reproductive organs at a young age. regulates the metabolism of proteins, fats, carbohydrates and the mineral balance of the body. It may act directly or indirectly through the insulin-related somatomedin. The impact on the mineral balance is conditioned by the increased absorption of calcium from the intestines and the retention of electrolytes in the system, i.e., potassium, phosphates and sodium. It also increases the metabolic activity of bone tissue within the epiphyseal cartilages during the growth of long bones (Ranke et al., 2018).

It works anabolic by stimulating the uptake of amino acids by cells and protein synthesis, while inhibiting proteolysis, resulting in a positive nitrogen balance. The lipolytic action is based on the activation of hormone-dependent lipase, fatty acids (FA – free acids) are released from the reservoirs of adipose tissue, it is worth noting that it is inhibited in the presence of insulin. The consequence of the lipolytic effect is the ketogenic effect – an increase in the concentration of FFA, an increase in the uptake of FFA by liver and muscle cells, and oxidation of free fatty acids by these cells. It also has a hyperglycemic effect, but much less than glucagon or adrenaline. It consists in inhibiting the uptake of glucose from the blood by cells of skeletal muscles and the liver, and thus reducing its use. In addition, it enhances the processes of glucose release from the liver, but it is not associated with increased glycogenolysis, as after the administration of somatropin, the level of glycogen increases, which imposes the conclusion that it has a stimulating effect on gluconeogenesis. GH also reduces the sensitivity of skeletal muscle cells and adipose tissue to insulin – it has anti-insulin and daibetogenic properties. Somatomedins, on the other hand, have the opposite effect, insulin-like, such as: increasing lipid synthesis and glucose consumption, inhibiting the effect of adrenaline on lipolysis. Additionally, GH binds to the prolactin receptor, showing a trophic effect on mammary gland cells (Siebert et al., 2018).

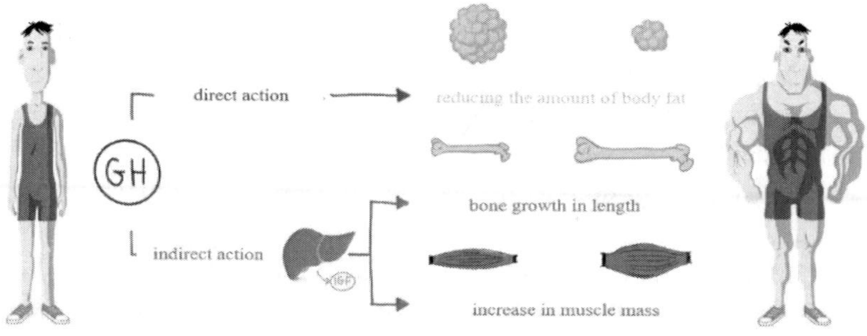

Figure 1. The mode of action of growth hormone [Own elaboration].

Adenoma of eosinophils in the anterior pituitary gland leads to acromegaly in adults, and gigantism in adolescent children. Symptoms of acromegaly are local bone growth, mainly of the skull, including the mandible. It also causes premature fusion of the epiphyseal cartilages of long bones – no linear growth. Gigantism, on the other hand, is characterized by an excessive linear growth of long bones and the accompanying underdevelopment of the gonads, or delayed fusion of the epigastric cartilages. Pituitary dwarfism is caused by a deficiency of gonadotrophins, and reduced or no GH secretion. The idiopathic origin of this pathology may be related to a tumor within the Turkish saddle and post-inflammatory or post-traumatic lesions. Symptoms are growth inhibition at normal body weight, usually visible in 2-3 years of age, although growth is disturbed in the following years as well. Sexual maturation is also impaired in older children. Mental development is normal (Siebert et al., 2018).

W Growth hormone is the most important factor in regulating weight gain in the body. Its deficiency leads to the development of severely disabling dysfunctions, such as dwarfism, while its too high concentration may lead to acromegaly or gigantism. In addition to the effects of this hormone visible to the naked eye, there are many others, such as the effect on the metabolism of connective tissues, which in the case of bone tissue is also associated with the regulation of water and electrolyte balance. The norms of growth hormone levels differ for adults and children: they range from about 1 to 12 ng / ml for adults and from about 10 to 30 ng / ml for children. Due to the fact that GH facilitates fat burning and influences the growth of muscle mass, growth hormone supplementation is usually interested in people practicing strength, body and endurance sports. The use of injections or tablets containing growth hormone is also recommended by bodybuilders on internet forums, but it is not indifferent to the body. GH used for a long time may lead to hypoglycaemia and an increase in the concentration of free fatty acids in the plasma, and in extreme cases even to the development of acromegaly. Taking supplements containing the so-called growth hormone precursors and an appropriate diet that increases the synthesis of somatropin in the body.

References

Aguiar-Oliveira MH, Bartke A. Growth Hormone Deficiency: Health and Longevity. *Endocr. Rev.* 2019;40(2):575-601.

Caicedo D, Díaz O, Devesa P, Devesa J. Growth Hormone (GH) and Cardiovascular System. *Int. J. Mol. Sci.* 2018;19(1):290.

Martínez-Moreno C G, Arámburo C. Growth hormone (GH) and synaptogenesis. *Vitam. Horm. 2020*;114:91-123.

Ranke M B, Wit J M. Growth hormone - past, present and future. *Nat. Rev. Endocrinol.* 2018 May;14(5):285-300.

Siebert D M, Rao A L. The Use and Abuse of Human Growth Hormone in Sports. *Sports Health.* 2018;10(5):419-426.

Chapter 10

Luteinizing Hormone (LH)

Matylda Mikołajczyk, Dorota Bartusik-Aebisher* and David Aebisher

Medical College of The University of Rzeszów, Rzeszów, Poland

Abstract

Luteinizing hormone belongs to the group of hormones with a similar peptide and to the group of gonadotropic hormones. Luteinizing hormone is necessary for the proper functioning of the body of both women and men. Lutropin has clinical application in assisted reproductive techniques and *in vitro* fertilization. Luteinizing hormone is usually administered by subcutaneous injection in a cyclic and stepwise manner. Like every hormone, it has a certain activation mechanism and therefore its action is possible only after binding to the receptor. It is a steroid hormone, the synthesis of which requires a precursor in the form of lipids. This hormone is extremely important in maintaining a proper menstrual cycle, which is a determinant of a woman's health and fertility. As the latest research has shown, lutropin supplementation seems to be helpful in getting pregnant through artificial *in vitro* fertilization. Certainly, the full potential of luteinizing hormone has yet to be discovered.

Keywords: luteinizing hormone (LH), lutropin/choriogonadotropin receptor (LHR), protein kinase A (PKA), protein kinase C (PKC), hypoxia-induced factors (HIF)

* Corresponding Author's Email: dbartusikaebisher@ur.edu.pl.

In: The Biochemical Guide to Hormones
Editor: David Aebisher
ISBN: 979-8-88697-492-8

Luteinizing hormone belongs to the group of hormones with a similar peptide structure called glycoproteins and to the group of gonadotropic hormones. It is secreted by the gonadotropic cells of the anterior pituitary gland. Lutein secretion takes place through stimulation by the hypothalamic gonadoliberin. LH influences the maturation process of the ovarian follicles. In the middle of the menstrual cycle, a surge of luteinizing hormone triggers ovulation, which releases the second-order oocyte into the banks of the fallopian tube. Another function of LH is to stimulate the production of progesterone in the ovaries by stimulating the epithelial cells and luteinized cells of the granule layer, which is necessary to ensure the proper conditions for the implantation of the fertilized oocyte (Arroyo et al. 2020). It is also responsible for luteinization of the corpus luteum, which means turning granular cells into lutein cells. In men, LH stimulates the synthesis of testosterone by Leydig cells in the testicles' seminiferous tubules. Lutropin has clinical application in assisted reproductive techniques and *in vitro* fertilization. So far, forms derived from urine (menotropin, Menopur) and recombinant (lutropin alfa: Luveris) human LH have been developed, but at the moment there is a problem with their availability. Luteinizing hormone is usually administered by subcutaneous injection in a cyclic and stepwise manner. These agents should be dosed with due caution and only under the supervision of a specialist physician best experienced in the treatment of infertility and hypogonadism (Deswal et al. 2019).

Like every hormone, it has a certain activation mechanism and therefore its action is possible only after binding to the receptor. It is a steroid hormone, the synthesis of which requires a precursor in the form of lipids. The discharge of lutropin stimulates the follicular cells to accumulate precursors in the form of cholesterol-containing lipid droplets. Without normal function of the lutropin/choriogonadotropin receptor (LHR) receptor, reproduction cannot take place. When LHR is not working properly, ovulation does not occur in women, and Leydig cells do not develop properly in men. Furthermore, since LHR is needed to maintain the high levels of progesterone needed to maintain pregnancy in the first trimester, disrupting LHR function during pregnancy would have dire consequences. For many years, LHR was thought to be localized only in gonadal cells. In the nucleus, the LHR is believed to be confined to Leydig cells. In the ovary, LHR is expressed in epithelial cells, interstitial cells, and differentiated granular and luteal cells (Duffy et al. 2019).

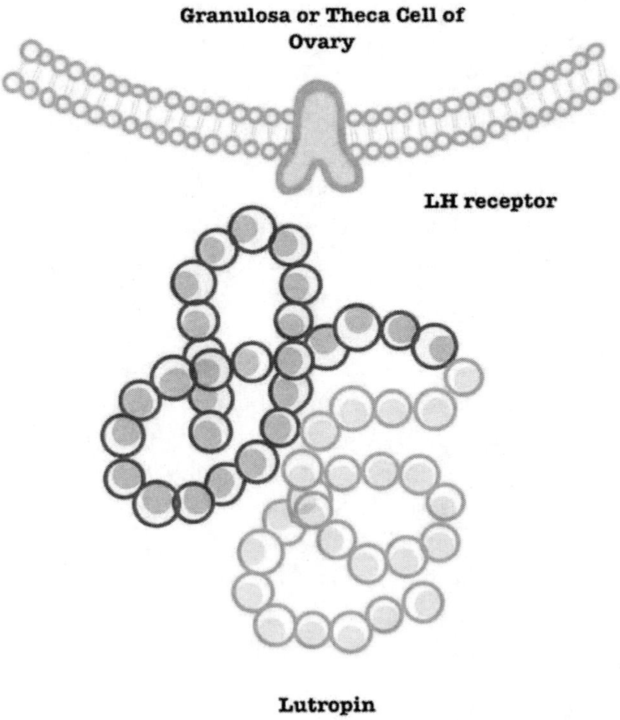

Figure 1. The molecule of lutropin and the hormone receptor found in the cell membrane of the ovarian granulosa cells or follicular cells.

In recent decades, the complexity of the signaling pathways triggered by pulses of the luteinizing hormone has come to light. Several laboratory studies have shown that LH activates a complex network of intracellular signaling cascades in pre-circulatory vesicles, including protein kinase A (PKA), protein kinase C (PKC) and protein kinase C (PKC), phosphatidylinositol 3-kinase. (PI3K), a tyrosine kinase mediated pathway and their respective downstream MAPKs. Lutropin is known to activate adenylate cyclase and increase intracellular cAMP as the main intracellular signaling molecule. Increased cAMP levels lead to cAMP-dependent PKA activation, which in turn activates the cAMP response factor binding protein (CREB). It is widely believed that this intracellular signaling (PKA) pathway is the major pathway mediating LH/hCG activity in the pre-ovulatory follicle. Specific transcription factors activated or induced by an increase in LH in the follicles directly regulate the transcription of various genes that induce specific effects related to tissue remodeling, angiogenesis and inflammatory response – such as hypoxia-induced factors (HIF), CEBPA and CEBPB, and base binders (RUNX1 and RUNX2), homologues of protein receptor 1 (NR5A20 and nuclear recptor 1 (NR1P1) (Mäkelä et al. 2020).

The effect of LH supplementation on the results of *in vitro* fertilization (IVF) has been assessed in several areas. For example, with a gonadotropin releasing hormone (GnRH) agonist, endogenous LH levels are very low in the late stimulation phase due to pituitary desensitization. Additionally, approximately 50% of patients undergo IVF/cytoplasmic injection into the cytoplasm (ICSI) using LH-GnRH agonist deficiency. Therefore, it seems reasonable that LH supplementation is beneficial for IVF/ICSI outcomes. However, it is still debatable whether LH supplementation at the end of the follicular phase can increase pregnancy and implantation rates, or reduce miscarriage rates. Studies have shown that LH supplementation not only improves the quality of the embryo, but also increases the pregnancy rate in women with poor ovarian reserve. Several studies have been carried out to evaluate the role of LH supplementation in the early phase of follicle growth. It has been shown that LH may increase the sensitivity of granulosa cells to FSH by increasing androgen synthesis in the early phase of folliculogenesis. However, due to the relatively small sample size, these studies were not sufficient for the pregnancy rate as the primary endpoint and did not provide conclusive information on the benefit of recombinant primary LH (rLH) dose in patients undergoing IVF/ICSI (Peter Dennis et al. 2020).

Luteinizing hormone is necessary for the proper functioning of the body of both women and men. Without adequate LH levels, ovulation will not be possible through the so-called lutropin release, and the ovaries will not be adequately stimulated to produce progesterone. This will cause problems with getting pregnant in women trying to conceive. This hormone is extremely important in maintaining a proper menstrual cycle, which is a determinant of a woman's health and fertility. In men, the deficiency of the luteinizing hormone will impair the synthesis of testosterone, which has various unfavorable consequences, including the weakening of the spermatogenesis process. However, in addition to the appropriate level and synthesis of the hormone, in order for it to fulfill its functions in the body, it is necessary for this protein to bind to the receptor, then the hormone can function properly. The proper level of the gonadoliberin hormone secreted by the hypothalamus is of course necessary for the proper synthesis of lutropin, thanks to which the hypothalamic-pituitary-ovarian axis is maintained, which regulates the synthesis of these hormones by feedback. As the latest research has shown, lutropin supplementation seems to be helpful in getting pregnant through artificial *in vitro* fertilization. Certainly, the full potential of luteinizing hormone has yet to be discovered.

References

Arroyo A, Kim B, Yeh J. Luteinizing Hormone Action in Human Oocyte Maturation and Quality: Signaling Pathways, Regulation, and Clinical Impact. *Reprod Sci*. 2020 Jun;27(6):1223-1252.

Deswal R, Nanda S, Dang AS. Association of Luteinizing hormone and LH receptor gene polymorphism with susceptibility of Polycystic ovary syndrome. *Syst. Biol. Reprod. Med.* 2019 Oct;65(5):400-408.

Duffy DM, Ko C, Jo M, Brannstrom M, Curry TE. Ovulation: Parallels with Inflammatory Processes. *Endocr. Rev*. 2019 Apr 1;40(2):369-416.

Mäkelä R, Leinonen A, Suominen T. Analysis of luteinizing hormone (LH): Validation of a commercial ELISA kit for LH analysis and quantification in doping control samples. *Drug Test Anal.* 2020 Feb;12(2):239-246.

Peter Dennis L, Nocillado J, Palma P, Amagai T, Soyano K, Elizur A. Development of a giant grouper Luteinizing Hormone (LH) Enzyme-Linked Immunosorbent Assay (ELISA) and its use towards understanding sexual development in grouper. *Gen. Comp Endocrinol.* 2020 Sep 15;296:113542.

Chapter 11

Follicle-Stimulating Hormone (FSH)

Maria Superson, Dorota Bartusik-Aebisher*
and David Aebisher
Medical College of The University of Rzeszów, Poland

Abstract

Follicle-stimulating hormone (FSH) is a tropic hormone and has a peptide structure. It consists of 207 amino acids that make up two subunits – alpha and beta. The decrease in serum FSH levels causes the smaller follicles in a given cohort to atresia because they do not have enough FSH sensitivity to survive. FSH levels are measured in International Units (IU). High FSH levels indicate that there is a lack of normal restrictive gonadal feedback, leading to unrestricted FSH production in the pituitary gland. High FSH may contribute to postmenopausal osteoporosis and cardiovascular disease. FSH is widely used in the treatment of infertility, mainly in ovarian hyperstimulation under the IVF method (in vitro). Sometimes it is also used to induce ovulation in the case of anovulation.

Keywords: follicle-stimulating hormone, luteinizing hormone (LH), gonadotropin releasing hormone (GnRH), glandular, International Units (IU)

It is a tropic hormone, and therefore secreted by the cells of the anterior pituitary gland. It has a peptide structure. It consists of 207 amino acids that

* Corresponding Author's Email: dbartusikaebisher@ur.edu.pl.

In: The Biochemical Guide to Hormones
Editor: David Aebisher
ISBN: 979-8-88697-492-8

make up two subunits – alpha and beta. The secretion of follicle stimulating hormone is controlled by the hypothalamic releasing factor follicle-releasing factor (FSH-RH). FSH secretion is also controlled by a feedback mechanism with the participation of estradiol (Saadia et al., 2020).

It interacts with the luteinizing hormone (LH), stimulating the maturation of ovarian follicles and the production of estrogen in ovarian follicle granular cells. It also increases the activity of aromatase, an enzyme whose function is to convert androgens to estrogens. In men, it controls the function of the testicles. Stimulates spermatogenesis – stimulates sperm-forming epithelium and reduces apoptosis during the first wave of spermatogenesis. FSH contributes to the initiation and maintenance of spermatogenesis, but is not essential. It has been proven that in the absence of spermatogenesis, the efficiency of this process is reduced. Folliculotropin in men also causes enlargement of the seminal tubes, and also stimulates the production of androgen binding protein (this protein is crucial in the proper functioning of testosterone). In women, the menstrual cycle and its individual phases have a particular impact on the secretion of this hormone (Saadia et al., 2020).

FSH is excreted from the human body in the urine. Increased levels of FSH in the blood and urine can be observed in both men and women in the menopausal period, which is caused by the decline of the hormonal activity of the gonads. FSH is a 35.5 kDa glycoprotein heterodimer. Its structure is similar to that of luteinizing hormone (LH), thyroid stimulating hormone (TSH) and human chorionic gonadotrophin (hCG). The alpha subunits of the LH, FSH, TSH and hCG glycoproteins are identical and consist of 96 amino acids, while the beta subunits are different. Both subunits are essential for biological activity. FSH has a beta 111 amino acid subunit (FSH β) which confers a specific biological action on it and is responsible for its interaction with the follicle stimulating hormone receptor. The sugar part of the hormone is covalently bound to asparagine and consists of N-acetylgalactosamine, mannose, N-acetylglucosamine, galactose, and sialic acid (Kourbanhoussen et al., 2022).

In humans, the alpha subunit gene can be located at the cytogenetic site 6q14.3. It is expressed in two types of cells, in particular the anterior pituitary basophils. The beta subunit FSH gene is located on chromosome 11p13 and is expressed in gonadotrophic pituitary cells under the control of GnRH, inhibin inhibited and stimulated by activin. FSH regulates the development, growth, maturation and reproductive processes in the human body. In both men and women, FSH stimulates the maturation of primary germ cells (Kourbanhoussen et al., 2022).

As previously mentioned, in men, FSH activates Sertoli cells to secrete androgen binding proteins (ABP), regulated by a negative inhibin feedback mechanism in the anterior pituitary gland. Activation of Sertoli cells by FSH supports spermatogenesis and stimulates the secretion of inhibin B. FSH further stimulates primary spermatocytes to undergo first meiosis division to form secondary spermatocytes. In women, as inhibin B levels increase, FSH levels decline in the late follicular phase. Towards the end of the luteal phase, there is a slight increase in FSH which is likely to play a role in starting the next ovulatory cycle (Fatemi et al., 2021).

The control of FSH release from the pituitary gland is unknown. Low-frequency gonadotropin releasing hormone (GnRH) pulses increase FSH mRNA levels in rats, but are not directly correlated with increases in circulating FSH. GnRH has been shown to play an important role in FSH secretion, and the detachment of the hypothalamus and pituitary leads to the cessation of FSH secretion. Administration of GnRH leads to a return of FSH secretion. FSH undergoes estrogen feedback from the gonads via the hypothalamic-pituitary-gonadal axis.

FSH stimulates the growth and recruitment of immature follicles in the ovary. In early (small) antral follicles, FSH is the main survival factor that protects small antral follicles (2-5 mm in diameter in humans) from apoptosis (the programmed death of the somatic cells of the follicle and the oocyte). During the transition period between the luteal follicles, the serum concentration of progesterone and estrogen (mainly estradiol) decreases and no longer inhibits FSH release, finally reaching the FSH peak around the third day (the first day is the first day of menstruation). The number of small antral follicles is usually sufficient to produce sufficient inhibin B to lower the serum FSH level (Fatemi et al., 2021).

In addition, there is evidence that the gonadotropin suppressive factor produced by small vesicles in the first half of the follicular phase reduces the amplitude of pulsatile luteinizing hormone (LH) secretion, thus providing a more favorable environment for follicle growth and preventing premature luteinisation (Casarini et al., 2020).

As a woman approaches perimenopause, the number of small antral follicles involved in each cycle decreases and, consequently, insufficient amount of inhibin B is produced to completely lower FSH levels. As a consequence, the serum FSH level begins to increase. Eventually, the level of FSH becomes so high that FSH receptors are degraded, and after the menopause, any remaining small secondary vesicles are devoid of FSH or LH receptors.

When the follicle is 8-10 mm in diameter, it begins to release large amounts of estradiol. Usually in humans only one follicle becomes dominant and survives to grow to a size of 18-3 mm and ovulate, while the remaining follicles undergo atresia. The sharp increase in the production of oestradiol by the dominant follicle (presumably with a decrease in the gonadotropin suppression factor) has a positive effect on the hypothalamus and pituitary gland. Rapid GnRH bursts take place and a burst of LH occurs (Ayman et al., 2021).

An increase in serum estradiol levels reduces the production of FSH by inhibiting the production of GnRH in the hypothalamus. The decrease in serum FSH levels causes the smaller follicles in a given cohort to atresia because they do not have enough FSH sensitivity to survive. Sometimes two follicles accidentally reach the 10 mm stage at the same time, and since both are equally sensitive to FSH, both survive and grow in a low FSH environment. Therefore, there can be two ovulations in one cycle, which can lead to pregnancy with dizygotic twins. Follicle stimulating hormone is usually measured early in the follicular phase of the menstrual cycle, usually between days 3 and 5 from the last menstrual period. During this time, estradiol and progesterone levels are at their lowest levels throughout the menstrual cycle. At the same time, FSH levels are referred to as basal FSH levels to distinguish them from levels that are increased in the period of impending ovulation (Casarini et al., 2020).

FSH levels are measured in International Units (IU). For FSH tested in human urine, one IU is defined as the amount of FSH whose activity corresponds to 0.11388 mg of pure human FSH in urine. For recombinant FSH, one IU corresponds to approximately 0.065 to 0.075 μg of "filled by weight" product. In women, FSH levels are typically low in childhood, high after the menopause. High FSH levels indicate that there is a lack of normal restrictive gonadal feedback, leading to unrestricted FSH production in the pituitary gland. High FSH may contribute to postmenopausal osteoporosis and cardiovascular disease (Ayman et al., 2021).

If a high level of FSH occurs during the childbearing period, it is pathological. In the greatest number of cases it indicates reduced fertility or complete sterility.

Reduced FSH secretion may result in gonadal failure (hypogonadism). This condition, in men, is usually manifested by a failure to produce a normal sperm count. In women, however, the cessation of reproductive cycles is often observed. FSH is widely used in the treatment of infertility, mainly in ovarian hyperstimulation under the IVF method (in vitro). Sometimes it is also used to induce ovulation in the case of anovulation. Elevated levels of FSH receptor have been detected in the endothelium of tumor blood vessels in a very wide range of solid tumors. FSH binding is believed to increase neovascularization by at least two mechanisms – one in the VEGF pathway and one independent of VEGF – associated with umbilical cord vessel development under physiological conditions. This demonstrates the possible use of FSH and FSH receptor antagonists as anti-tumor angiogenesis.

References

Ayman A H, Anas A O, Yasser A A, Masad A M, Abdullah A S, Mazen A, Salih A G, Saad A S, Abdulraheem A, AbdulRhman A G, Al-Gthami O. Levels of Follicle Stimulating Hormone (FSH), Luteinizing Hormone (LH), Testosterone and Prolactin at Moderate Altitude Inhabitant Male. *Pak. J. Biol. Sci.* 2021; 24(2): 188-192.

Casarini L, Crépieux P, Reiter E, Lazzaretti C, Paradiso E, Rochira V, Brigante G, Santi D, Simoni M. FSH for the Treatment of Male Infertility. *Int. J. Mol. Sci.* 2020; 21(7): 2270.

Fatemi H, Bilger W, Denis D, Griesinger G, La Marca A, Longobardi S, Mahony M, Yin X, D'Hooghe T. Dose adjustment of follicle-stimulating hormone (FSH) during ovarian stimulation as part of medically-assisted reproduction in clinical studies: a systematic review covering 10 years (2007-2017). *Reprod. Biol. Endocrinol.* 2021; 19(1): 68.

Kourbanhoussen K, Joncas F H, D Wallis C J, Hovington H, Dagenais F, Fradet Y, Guillemette C, Lacombe L, Toren P. Follicle-stimulating hormone (FSH) levels prior to prostatectomy are not related to long-term oncologic or cardiovascular outcomes for men with prostate cancer. *Asian J. Androl.* 2022; 24(1): 21-25.

Saadia Z. Follicle Stimulating Hormone (LH: FSH) Ratio in Polycystic Ovary Syndrome (PCOS) - Obese vs. Non- Obese Women. *Med. Arch.* 2020; 74(4): 289-293.

Chapter 12

Analogs of Prolactin

Katarzyna Jucha, Dorota Bartusik-Aebisher*
and David Aebisher
Medical College of The University of Rzeszów, Poland

Abstract

The main form of prolactin found in the pituitary gland is prolactin with a mass of 23 kDa. The 16 kDa prolactin is a product of the enzymatic activity of kallikrein and is believed to be due to proteolytic cleavage. Prolactin can be detected in the cells of the mammary gland epithelium during lactation, as well as in the milk itself, which comes from the pituitary gland and reaches the mammary gland through circulation. In addition to the uptake of prolactin from the blood, the mammary epithelial cells of lactating animals are capable of self-synthesizing prolactin. Prolactin is a common mediator of the immunoneuroendocrine network where the nervous, endocrine and immune systems communicate with each other. Recent studies show that prolactin stimulates mitogenesis in both normal T cells and the Nb2 lymphoma cell line (1622). Since in most cases the secretory response of prolactin (i.e., stimulation or inhibition) differs with the type of stress, a uniform mechanism of the influence of stress conditions on secretion of this hormone cannot be described.

Keywords: prolactin, tumor necrosis factor (TNF), Sjögren's syndrome, systemic lupus erythematosus (SLE), rheumatoid arthritis (RA)

---

* Corresponding Author's Email: dbartusikaebisher@ur.edu.pl.

In: The Biochemical Guide to Hormones
Editor: David Aebisher
ISBN: 979-8-88697-492-8

Prolactin is a peptide hormone found in all vertebrate animals. The place defined as the production center marks the angular cells of the anterior pituitary gland called lactotrophs. In addition, we can also show its presence in other tissues such as the placenta, intestine, brain and tissues belonging to the immune system. The production and secretion of this compound is regulated by a special inhibitory hormone called dopamine, secreted by the hypothalamus.

The age of the gene from which the family of three peptide hormones, which we include prolactin, is derived, is estimated at 400 million years. The hormone precursor – preprolactin consists of 227 amino acids, while the active form is composed of 199 amino acids. The lactotropic hormone is a protein with a molecular weight of about 23 kDa (Bernard et al., 2019).

Prolactin, also known as PRL, can undergo many post-translational modifications, which allow to regulate the current state of the organism by modifying the biological activity of the hormone, which contributes to regulating the influence exerted on target tissues. The most common function of prolactin is to stimulate lactation in women. Currently, we are able to identify over 300 functions of this compound, which can be broken down into six categories: osmoregulation, growth and development, metabolism, behavior, immunomodulation and reproduction. Recent studies have also proven the relationship between this hormone and the immune system in common cases of fighting parasitic infections, and its influence on the development of progressive rheumatic diseases (Borba et al., 2018).

The secretion of PRL is tightly regulated by the neurotransmitter dopamine, which binds to specific type 2 dopamine receptors in the pituitary gland, resulting in a reduction in the secretion of this hormone. Prolactin is a hormone secreted in a strictly defined circadian rhythm. Frequent repetitive night work can disturb the circadian rhythm and therefore has the potential to modify the rhythm of prolactin secretion (Cabrera-Reyes et al., 2017).

The concentration of prolactin in the blood may also increase through a positive feedback mechanism between the immune system and the neurohormonal system after intravenous administration of specific pro-inflammatory cytokines. Normal PRL concentration is lower than 20 ng / ml in women and usually lower than 15 ng / ml in men. The increase in the concentration of this hormone is usually the result of stress or consumed a large meal and does not exceed 30 ng / ml. Interestingly, an increase in the concentration of PRL is also observed as a result of smoking tobacco with a high nicotine content. However, during the research, it was possible to observe a decrease in the concentration of prolactin in the case of administering even a small amount of cocaine to a person who is highly addicted to this substance. The most common activity of the PRL is the stimulation of the development of the lobular-alveolar part of the mammary gland and the induction and maintenance of lactation in breastfeeding women. Additionally, the role of prolactin in maintaining proper calcium metabolism in pregnant women should be taken into account. Increasing the concentration of PRL in the blood during pregnancy stimulates the reabsorption of calcium in the kidneys and increases its absorption in the small intestine, which is particularly important due to the increased demand for this element in a given period of the woman's body. Moreover, it was found that prolactin causes an increase in transcellular absorption, which takes place mainly in the duodenum, in the brush border of the enterocyte (Carretero et al., 2019).

This hormone also has a verified activity based on the stimulation and production of progesterone in the corpus luteum. A less known function of the PRL is its participation in regulating the developing, normal immune response. Its main task focuses on the process of proliferation and differentiation of the immune system cells and the angiogenesis process in the thymus. PRL stimulates the proliferation of T and B lymphocytes, stimulates the secretion by cells of immunoglobulins and cytokines, e.g., IL-1b, IL-6, tumor necrosis factor (TNF) and interferon-g. Many studies indicate the participation of PRL in the pathogenesis of various autoimmune diseases, which include systemic connective tissue diseases, including systemic lupus erythematosus (SLE), rheumatoid arthritis (RA), Sjögren's syndrome, systemic sclerosis, rheumatic polymyalgia and seronegative arthritis. There is also a clear relationship between the PRL and the course and activity of PsA. In recent years, when psoriatic arthritis was diagnosed, administration of non-bromocriptine was started – a drug whose action is to lower the concentration of the hormone prolactin. During this experiment, it was possible to observe the alleviation of joint and skin symptoms, which translated into an improvement in the clinical picture of the disease. The hormone prolactin in the case of men observed during clinical trials is responsible for regulating the processes related to sexual activity, and the secretion of PRL in men is strictly regulated by many other hormones, drugs, and current physiological situations (Phillipps et al., 2020).

In the human genome, a single gene on chromosome 6 codes for prolactin. This gene is 10 kb in size and consists of 5 exons and 4 introns. Transcription of the prolactin gene is regulated by two independent promoter regions. The 5,000-bp proximal region drives pituitary-specific expression, while the more upstream promoter region is responsible for extra-pituitary expression. The main form of prolactin found in the pituitary gland is prolactin with a mass of 23 kDa, it has been possible to characterize its various variants in humans. The prolactin variants may result from primary transcript alternative splicing, proteolytic cleavage, and other post-translational modifications of the amino acid chain. Indeed, evidence suggesting the existence of an alternatively spliced 137 amino acid variant of prolactin has been reported in the anterior pituitary. In addition, it was assumed that alternative splicing while preserving introns was also possible, although it is not considered a major source of prolactin variants, however. The 16 kDa prolactin is a product of the enzymatic activity of kallikrein and is believed to be due to proteolytic cleavage. Kallikrein is an estrogen-induced, trypsin-like serine protease that is found in the Golgi cisterns and in the secretory granules of lactotrophs. The first observation confirming the production of prolactin in the brain was made by Fuxe and associates who found prolactin immunoreactivity at the axon terminals of the hypothalamus. It was then validated in the hippocampus, amygdala, septum, brainstem, cerebellum, spinal cord, choroid plexuses, and periventricular organs, among others. Some well-known factors that stimulate the secretion of pituitary prolactin, such as ovarian steroids, are responsible for the regulation of prolactin synthesis in the hypothalamus. About 33% of the immunoreactive prolactin neurons in the medial basal hypothalamus can be labeled with estradiols, suggesting that these neurons have estrogen receptors. Performing an ovariectomy lowers the prolactin content in the hypothalamus, while estrogen replacement increases it. Among the known hypophysiotropic factors, angiotensin II stimulates the release of prolactin from fragments of the hypothalamus, and intracerebral injection of vasoactive intestinal peptide increases the amount of hypothalamic prolactin mRNA. However, other recognized stimulants of prolactin secretion from the pituitary gland, such as TRH, have no effect. Of course, most of the mechanisms involved in prolactin release in the hypothalamus have not yet been thoroughly investigated. Prolactin can be detected in the cells of the mammary gland epithelium during lactation, as well as in the milk itself, which comes from the pituitary gland and reaches the mammary gland through circulation. It can therefore be concluded that part of the prolactin found in milk is taken up and not produced by the cells of the mammary gland epithelium. This was confirmed in studies when a significant amount of radiolabelled hormone introduced into the circulation appeared in the milk. Most likely, prolactin reaches the milk by first passing through the basal membrane of the breast epithelial cells, attaching to a specific protein binding it in the breast epithelial cell, and is finally transported by exocytosis through the terminal membrane into the lumen of the alveolus.

In addition to the uptake of prolactin from the blood, the mammary epithelial cells of lactating animals are capable of self-synthesizing prolactin. The presence of prolactin mRNA has been reported, as well as the synthesis of immunoreactive prolactin by the mammary epithelial cells of lactating rats. It is possible that de novo synthesis of prolactin in the breast requires a systemic trophic factor as both prolactin and immunoreactive prolactin mRNAs decline within 24-48 h in mammary explants. The mammary gland may also undergo post-translational processing of the hormone. In both human and rat milk, the number of prolactin variants far exceeds the number of variants found in serum. Indeed, the mammary gland is the site of an important 16-kDa variant of prolactin. While prolactin, produced locally by breast epithelial cells, promotes proliferation, the 16-kDa split prolactin variant inhibits local angiogenesis, making this proteolytic step a possible target for breast cancer research. Prolactin is a common mediator of the immunoneuroendocrine network where the nervous, endocrine and immune systems communicate with each other. Prolactin plays an important role in the regulation of the humoral and cellular immune response in both physiological and pathological conditions, such as autoimmune diseases previously considered.

The earliest evidence that prolactin plays a role in the immune response came in 1972 when it was shown that exogenous prolactin enhanced thymic function in prolactin-deficient dwarf mice. Shortly thereafter, it was proved that hypophyctomy or inhibition of prolactin secretion with bromocriptine led to a decline in humoral or cellular immunity that could be reversed by treatment with the exogenous form of the hormone. Recent studies show that prolactin stimulates mitogenesis in both normal T cells and the Nb2 lymphoma cell line (1622). It should come as no surprise that prolactin affects lymphocytes since prolactin-R has been detected on human peripheral lymphocytes and their mRNA expression is regulated by prolactin itself. Moreover, the effects of the hormone on lymphocytes may include the interleukin IL-2. Interestingly, the nucleus may be behind the site where prolactin modifies the action of IL-2. Prolactin is also essential for mitogen-stimulated lymphocyte proliferation. Nb2 cells, derived from immature T lymphocytes, are closely dependent on the mitogenic activity of prolactin. This property served as the basis for a highly sensitive, specific prolactin bioassay. Despite these discoveries, we cannot define the function of prolactin in the process of hematopoiesis.

The secretion of prolactin is largely related to external factors. Secretion is greatly influenced by the change in the intensity of light acting on an individual related to circadian rhythms. In the case of long-term observation of the effect of high-intensity light on the test subject from selected species of rats used for the study, significant jumps in the secretion of this hormone depending on the time of day were observed. It is clear that prolactin secretion is dramatically influenced by "stress." Countless types of stress have been used to characterize this effect on prolactin secretion. These include, but are not limited to, ether stress, restraint stress, thermal stress, hemorrhage, social conflict (817), and even academic stress.

Since in most cases the secretory response of prolactin (i.e., stimulation or inhibition) differs with the type of stress, a uniform mechanism of the influence of stress conditions on secretion of this hormone cannot be described.

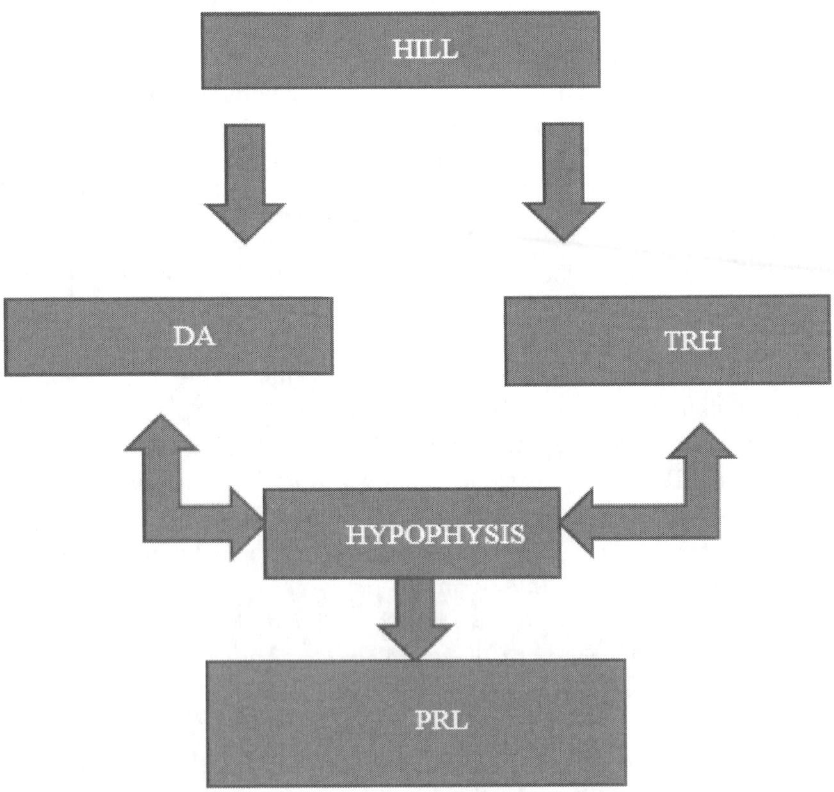

Figure 1. Feedback for the release of prolactin by the pituitary gland. [Own study].

References

Bernard V, Young J, Binart N. Prolactin - a pleiotropic factor in health and disease. *Nat. Rev. Endocrinol.* 2019;15(6):356-365.

Borba V V, Zandman-Goddard G, Shoenfeld Y. Prolactin and Autoimmunity. *Front. Immunol.* 2018;9:73.

Cabrera-Reyes EA, Limón-Morales O, Rivero-Segura NA, Camacho-Arroyo I, Cerbón M. Prolactin function and putative expression in the brain. *Endocrine.* 2017;57(2):199-213.

Carretero J, Sánchez-Robledo V, Carretero-Hernández M, Catalano-Iniesta L, García-Barrado MJ, Iglesias-Osma MC, Blanco E J. Prolactin system in the hippocampus. *Cell Tissue Res.* 2019;375(1):193-199.

Phillipps H R, Yip S H, Grattan D R. Patterns of prolactin secretion. *Mol. Cell Endocrinol.* 2020;502:110679.

Chapter 13

Thyroid Stimulating Hormone (TSH)

Marcelina Dymon, Izabela Kiebała, Dorota Bartusik-Aebisher[*] and David Aebisher
Medical College of The University of Rzeszów, Rzeszów, Poland

Abstract

Thyroid stimulating hormone (TSH), also known as thyroid stimulating hormone, is a hormone that stimulates the metabolism of virtually every tissue in the body. TSH is consisting of two subunits produced by the anterior pituitary gland. The primary target site of TSH action is the thyroid gland. These hormones affect the entire body, especially by affecting the body's metabolism, but also affect the functions of entire systems such as the cardiovascular system. Primary thyroid disease refers to problems arising from the thyroid gland itself. A problem with the thyroid gland may appear in the form of an overactive or underactive thyroid gland. The thyroid stimulating hormone is therefore a factor necessary to maintain homeostasis in the body.

Keywords: thyroid stimulating hormone, (TSH), subacute thyroiditis (SAT), triiodothyronine (T3), follicle stimulating hormone (FSH)

It's hard to say who first discovered and named the thyroid stimulating hormone. In fact, the answer spans many stories and many names. It is worth noting that before the start of specific studies in the 20th century on the effects of the anterior pituitary hormone, it was widely believed that this organ contained a thyroid stimulating substance. In 1910 there were reports of

[*] Corresponding Author's Email: dbartusikaebisher@ur.edu.pl.

In: The Biochemical Guide to Hormones
Editor: David Aebisher
ISBN: 979-8-88697-492-8

thyroid atrophy being observed after some pituitary surgeries. Key contributors to the development of this issue were two young biologists, Bennett M. Allen and Philip E. Smith, who in independent studies used tadpoles as an inexpensive model system because it was known (largely thanks to Allen) that the thyroid was essential for the tadpole to pass through. metamorphosis into a frog. Using a microscope, it was possible to relatively precisely remove the anterior pituitary glands of larval amphibians at some anatomically favorable stage of development, and then observe the subsequent biological effect in the structure of thyroid follicles. Both Allen and Smith conducted such experiments which gave quite similar results. Both noticed that many of the tadpoles developed thyroid follicular lesions with less colloid, which resulted, among other things, in that the tadpoles grew slowly, their legs did not enlarge, and the dark pigment grains in their skin shrank so that the animals turned a creamy silver color. color. Both researchers studied this phenomenon in other studies, extending their knowledge in this regard (Carty et al., 2017).

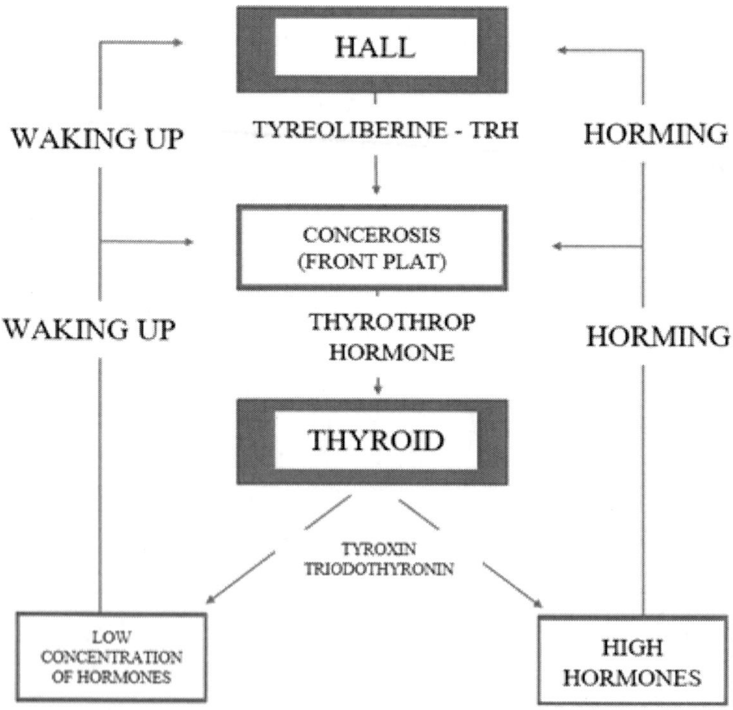

Figure 1. Diagram: How feedback works.

Another significant period in the understanding of TSH began in 1953, when ion exchange chromatography was used to prepare much purer preparations of TSH, but peptide sequencing attempts were unsuccessful. In the late 1950s, an improved technique of ion exchange chromatography led to cleaner TSH preparations with the recognition that TSH consists of 2 peptide chains. The following years brought fruitful results, in the understanding of the subunit structure of thyrotropic hormone, the peptide sequences of these subunits were determined. Subsequent advances by many people have led to a detailed molecular and physiological understanding of the very important hormone TSH. One of the applications of this knowledge was the production of recombinant human TSH, used in the diagnosis and therapy of, for example, thyroid cancer (Carty et al., 2017).

Hyroid stimulating hormone (TSH), also known as thyroid stimulating hormone, is a hormone that stimulates the metabolism of virtually every tissue in the body. This hormone is a glycoprotein produced by the thyroid stimulating cells of the anterior pituitary gland and regulates the endocrine functions of the thyroid gland.

TSH is made up of two subunits, alpha and beta:

- alpha, i.e., alpha chorionic gonadotropin, is virtually identical to the subunit of human chorionic gonadotrophin (hCG), follicle stimulating hormone (FSH) and luteinizing hormone (LH). The α-subunit is believed to be the effector region responsible for stimulation of adenylate cyclase (involved in the production of cAMP). The α chain consists of a 92 amino acid sequence.
- Beta (TSHB) is unique to TSH and therefore it determines its receptor specificity. The β chain consists of a sequence of 118 amino acids.

TSH stimulates the thyroid gland to secrete thyroxine (T4), but it has little effect on metabolism. Only thyroxine (T4) is converted into the active thyroid stimulating hormone triiodothyronine (T3). About 80% of this conversion occurs in the liver and the remaining 20% in the thyroid itself TSH is secreted throughout life, but it is especially high during periods of rapid growth and development, and in response to stress. Before TSH is released, the hypothalamus produces a hormone that releases thyrotropin (TRH), which stimulates the anterior pituitary gland to produce TSH. Somatostatin is a hormone with an opposite effect on the production of TSH secreted by the hypothalamus, because it reduces or inhibits its secretion. The secretion of TSH by the pituitary gland is regulated by the concentration of thyroid hormones (T3 and T4) in the blood. When T3 and T4 levels are low, TSH production is increased, while when T3 and T4 levels are high, TSH production is reduced. The presented dependency is an example of a negative feedback operation. Any disruption, for example, low TSH levels combined with low normal T4 can signal TSH pathology to TRH and central disease. Elevated inverted T3 (RT3) along with normal TSH values and low normal T3, T4 values, which are considered indicative of euthyroid disease syndrome (a medical term that means normal thyroid function based on hormone release criteria), you may also need to be tested for chronic subacute thyroiditis (SAT). Patients with a prior diagnosis of autoimmune thyroid disease who lack antibodies are suspected of developing SAT, even with normal TSH levels, as there is no known method of recovery from autoimmunity (Soh et al., 2019).

For the interpretation of laboratory results, it is important to recognize that TSH is released in a pulsatile manner (pulsatile secretion is a biochemical phenomenon observed in many different types of cells and tissues, in which products are secreted at regular intervals, including intercellular signaling molecules, i.e., hormones or neurotransmitters), which is a result of both the circadian rhythm and the ultradian rhythm of its serum concentrations (Jasim et al., 2018).

The TSH receptor is found mainly on the follicular cells of the thyroid gland. Thanks to its stimulation, the production and secretion of T3 and T4 increases, as a result of the stimulation of six stages of the synthesis of thyroid hormones:

1. Increased sodium iodide symporter (NIS) activity on the basolateral membrane of thyroid follicular cells, leading to an increase in intracellular sodium concentration.
2. Stimulating thyroglobulin iodination in the lumen of the follicle, thyroid hormone precursor protein.
3. Stimulating the conjugation of iodinated tyrosine residues. This produces thyroxine (T4) and triiodothyronine (T3), which remain attached to the thyroglobulin protein.
4. Increased endocytosis of iodinated thyroglobulin protein across the apical membrane back into the follicular cell.
5. Stimulation of the proteolysis of iodinated thyroglobulin to form free thyroxine (T4) and triiodothyronine (T3).
6. Secretion of thyroxine (T4) and triiodothyronine (T3) by the basolateral membrane of the follicular cells in order to enter the

circulation. This is due to an unknown mechanism (Wang et al., 2020).

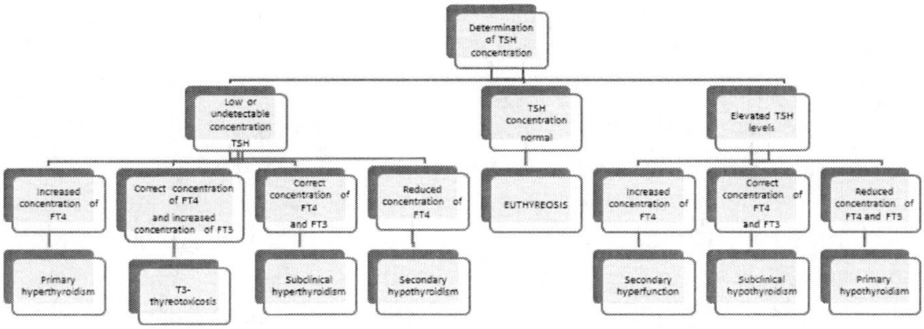

Figure 2. Scheme: Determination of TSH concentration.

For an adult, the range of TSH norms is from 0.32 to 5.0 mU/l. The level of FSH is influenced by age, sex and the method of determination used by the laboratory in which the test was performed, therefore it is very important to interpret the obtained test results on the basis of the range of standards set by the laboratory. The range of this hormone is different in women planning to start a family or in women who are already pregnant. When FSH levels exceed 2.5 mU/l, this is cause for concern and further tests must be carried out as soon as possible. FSH norms in pregnant women are as follows:

- I trimester - from 0.1 to 2.5 mIU/l,
- II trimester - from 0.1 to 3.0 mIU/l,
- III trimester - from 0.1 to 3.0 mIU/l.

However, in children immediately after birth, a normal TSH result is 19 mlU/l, during the first 10 weeks of a child's life, the TSH level ranges between 0.6-10 mlU/l, in children several years old 0.4-6.0 mlU/l and in adolescents, the norm is 0.4-5.0 mlU/l (Wang et al., 2020).

Increased FSH levels can mean that you have an underactive pituitary gland, an underactive thyroid gland (hypothyroidism), or Hashimoto's thyroiditis. Elevated TSH may also indicate that the ongoing L-thyroxine replacement therapy is insufficient and requires modification. In pregnant women, hypothyroidism can cause preterm labor or miscarriage. Hypothyroidism (and therefore a high level of TSH) can be diagnosed by observing symptoms. The most important ones include: constant feeling of cold, fatigue, drowsiness, joint pain, weight gain (without a reason), swelling of the face and neck, depression, water retention, menstrual disorders, headaches, muscle stiffness, problems with memory and concentration, drop in mood, decreased libido, impotence, exercise fatigue, dry and itchy skin, shortness of breath (Wong i et al., 2020).

A lowered TSH value may be due to the presence of thyroid diseases, such as Graves' disease, hyperthyroidism (hyperthyroidism), and toxic nodular goitre. The following symptoms may indicate the presence of TSH level in the blood below the norm: excessive sweating, mood changes and nervousness, uncontrolled weight loss, noticeable trembling of the hands and fingers, menstrual cycle disorders, shortness of breath and diarrhea. When the tested TSH level gives a result below or above the norm, and the patient still has disturbing symptoms, free thyroid hormones fT3 and fT4 are additionally tested:

- The norm of fT3 is 2.25-6 pmol/l
- The norm of fT4 is 10-25 pmol/l.

The cause may be Graves' disease, most often autoimmune, in which the body produces antibodies against thyroid cells, which stimulates the synthesis of thyroid hormones. Other causes of primary hyperthyroidism include thyroid nodules, postpartum thyroiditis, and subacute thyroiditis (Wong i et al., 2020). The cause of the disease is a disturbed secretion of the hormone TSH by the pituitary gland. The recommended test is the TRH test, which allows the differentiation of a pituitary adenoma from the resistance of the pituitary to thyroid hormones.

In this case, the fT3 should be determined and the TSH level should be analyzed with its level. Decreased TSH and fT3 in the norm – subclinical hyperthyroidism, which does not show clinical symptoms; decreased TSH and increased fT3 - T3-thyrotoxicosis, which is high blood levels of triiodothyronine which may be caused, for example, by treatment with thyroid hormones; decreased TSH and decreased fT3- low triiodothyronine syndrome, usually accompanied; myocardial infarction, extensive trauma, decreased TSH synthesis and peripheral fT3 metabolism (Jasim et al., 2018).

TSH is a peptide hormone, or more precisely, it is a glycoprotein consisting of two subunits, produced by the anterior pituitary gland. The primary target site of TSH action is the thyroid gland. TSH increases blood flow to the thyroid gland and stimulates hypertrophy and hyperplasia of thyroid follicular cells, influencing the growth of the thyroid gland. However, the most important function of this hormone is to stimulate the secretion of thyroid hormones by increasing iodine uptake, thyroglobulin synthesis and thyreoperoxidase activity. These hormones affect the entire body, especially by affecting the body's metabolism, but also affect the functions of entire systems such as the cardiovascular system. Primary thyroid disease refers to problems arising from the thyroid gland itself. In turn, secondary thyroid diseases refer to the central problems arising from the anterior pituitary gland, which indirectly affect the functioning of the thyroid gland. A problem with the thyroid gland may appear in the form of an overactive or underactive thyroid gland. The thyroid stimulating hormone is therefore a factor necessary to maintain homeostasis in the body.

References

Carty D. M., Doogan F., Welsh P., Dominiczak A. F., Delles C. Thyroid stimulating hormone (TSH) ≥2.5 mU/l in early pregnancy: Prevalence and subsequent outcomes. *Eur J Obstet Gynecol Reprod Biol.* 2017 Mar;210:366-369.

Jasim S., Gharib H. Thyroid and Aging. Endocr Pract. 2018 Apr;24(4):369-374.

Wang Y., Dong X., Fu C., Su M., Jiang F., Xu D., Li R., Qian J., Wang N., Chen Y., Jiang Q. Thyroid Stimulating Hormone (TSH) Is Associated With General and Abdominal Obesity: A Cohort Study in School-Aged Girls During Puberty in East China. *Front Endocrinol* (Lausanne). 2020 Sep 30;11:620.

Wong J. S. L., Selveindran N. M., Mohamed R. Z., Zain F. M., Anas S. S., Hong J. Y. H. Reference intervals for thyroid-stimulating hormone (TSH) and free thyroxine (FT4) in infants' day 14-30 of life and a comparison with other studies. J Pediatr Endocrinol Metab. 2020 Sep 25;33(9):1125-1132. Soh SB, Aw TC. Laboratory Testing in Thyroid Conditions - Pitfalls and Clinical Utility. *Ann Lab Med.* 2019 Jan;39(1):3-14.

Chapter 14

Erythropoietin

**Zuzanna Kawa, Dorota Bartusik-Aebisher*
and David Aebisher**
Medical College of The University of Rzeszów, Rzeszów, Poland

Abstract

Erythropoietin plays an important role in the human body, it takes part in hematopoietic processes, stimulating erythropoiesis in hypoxic states. The erythropoietin molecule consists of amino acids, carbohydrates and sialic acid residues, responsible for maintaining the proper activity and stability of the hormone. Erythropoietin in adults is produced in small amounts in the liver and to a large extent in the kidneys, specifically in the vascular endothelial cells surrounding the renal tubules in the cortex of this organ. In the pharmaceutical industry, for therapeutic purposes, recombinant human erythropoietin is used as a drug that stimulates the production of red blood cells in the bone marrow. Testing the level of erythropoietin is used to select the therapy in anemia and in the case of kidney diseases. The analysis of the results allows you to control the effectiveness of the implemented treatment, for example in the treatment of certain types of cancer. Monitoring the level of erythropoietin is also used in doping control among athletes. Carried out to break out the illegal use of doping substances.

Keywords: erythropoietin (EPO), hormone, cytokine, tissue hypoxia

---

* Corresponding Author's Email: dbartusikaebisher@ur.edu.pl.

In: The Biochemical Guide to Hormones
Editor: David Aebisher
ISBN: 979-8-88697-492-8

Erythropoietin (EPO) is a cytokine glycoprotein peptide hormone with a total mass of 18 kDa. It is made of 165 amino acids. 40% of it consists of carbohydrates, 11% of which are sialic acid residues that maintain the stability of the molecule. In utero, it is produced in the liver, and after birth, this function is to a greater extent taken over by the kidneys. The synthesis of erythropoietin is regulated by the influence of thyroid hormones and the presence of oxygen, which results in the inhibition of EPO production by an increase in oxygen concentration. In the human body, erythropoietin is responsible for controlling and regulating the synthesis, maturation and release of red blood cells from the bone marrow into the blood (erythropoiesis). It is used in the treatment of anemia caused by kidney failure, chemotherapy and radiotherapy. It improves muscle endurance, increases the motivation to undertake exercise. The correct level of the hormone is 5-30 mU/ml, no significant fluctuations in these values depending on gender are observed. The level is regulated by the daily cycle, higher values occur at night, lower values occur in the morning. Too low levels of erythropoietin result in the body not producing enough red blood cells, which can lead to anemia. Too high concentration of EPO results in an excess of erythrocytes in the blood, which increases its viscosity and can lead to hypertension and thrombosis. Increased values are also observed in the bodies of people whose oxygen demand is greater, i.e., pregnant women, smokers, suffering from heart and lung diseases, and people living in high mountain areas (Bhoopalan et al. 2020).

Research on the action and structure of erythropoietin began about 150 years ago. The first concerned the relationship between the increase in hematocrit and staying at high altitudes. The correlation was investigated by Paul Bert and Viault. In 1948, Eva Bonsdorff and Eeva Jalavisto conducted research on the humoral mechanism of erythropoiesis regulation. The results of these studies are considered groundbreaking. In 1957, the next breakthrough was the test results of Jacobson and a team of researchers who proved that the production of Epo takes place in an isolated, perfused kidney. Subsequent studies aimed at cloning the erythropoietin gene, which were successful in 1985 (Bhoopalan et al. 2020).

The erythropoietin molecule consists of amino acids, carbohydrates and sialic acid residues, responsible for maintaining the proper activity and stability of the hormone. The disulfide bonds are responsible for the stabilization of the secondary structure. It is a glycoprotein peptide hormone belonging to the group of cytokines. Erythropoietin receptors are proteins made up of 508 amino acids, 24 of which constitute the signal sequence. The hormone molecule is bound to the receptor by the N-terminal extracellular domain, the hydrophobic transmembrane domain and the intracellular cytoplasmic C-terminal domain. Receptors appear on the early progenitor cells of the erythropoietic series. Their number increases in the CFU-E stage, and then, decreases, the reticulocyte is already insensitive to the action of erythropoietin (Ehrenreich et al. 2020).

Erythropoietin in adults is produced in small amounts in the liver and to a large extent in the kidneys, specifically in the vascular endothelial cells surrounding the renal tubules in the cortex of this organ. In utero, synthesis takes place in the liver (Juul et al. 2020).

Erythropoietin stimulates the bone marrow to produce red blood cells, granulocytes and platelets. It works by stimulating the proliferation and differentiation of precursor cells into mature erythrocytes. Erythropoietin combines the features of a cytokine, due to the mechanism of action and structure, and of a hormone, due to the place of production and the role it plays in the body. It is a growth factor for the erythroblastic system. The site of its action is the bone marrow, which justifies it belongs to cytokines. It also exhibits hormone properties, as it is produced in the kidney outside its site of action, i.e., the bone marrow, from where it reaches the target cell through the bloodstream (Sakaguchi et al. 2019).

The hormone affects erythropoiesis and its deficiency, caused by, for example, kidney damage, causes apoptosis of many precursors of red blood cells. This can lead to the development of anemia. The lack of response to the hormone in the bone marrow caused by myeloid diseases can aggravate the condition (Sakaguchi et al. 2019).

The impulse for increased secretion is the reduction of oxygen content in the blood flowing through the renal arterioles. Tissue hypoxia is caused, for example, by high altitude living, chronic obstructive pulmonary disease, heart disease, sleep apnea, carbon monoxide poisoning and bleeding. The hormone is active for a short time and is quickly excreted from the body once the oxygen level in the blood is stabilized. The increased concentration of erythropoietin is also an effect of the activity of kidney cancer cells, liver and ovarian cancers, uterine fibroids and adenocortical adenomas (Shih et al. 2018).

The determination of the concentration of erythropoietin in the blood serum is used mainly in the diagnosis of anemia and polycythemia. This test is also performed in patients with renal failure and bone marrow suppression. In addition to its use in medicine, for example in the treatment of anemia, the substance is widely used as an illegal doping agent among competitive athletes. Thanks to its administration, the athlete's body produces more red blood cells, and the transport of oxygen to the muscles becomes more efficient.

This results in improved efficiency, endurance and increased strength (Shih et al. 2018).

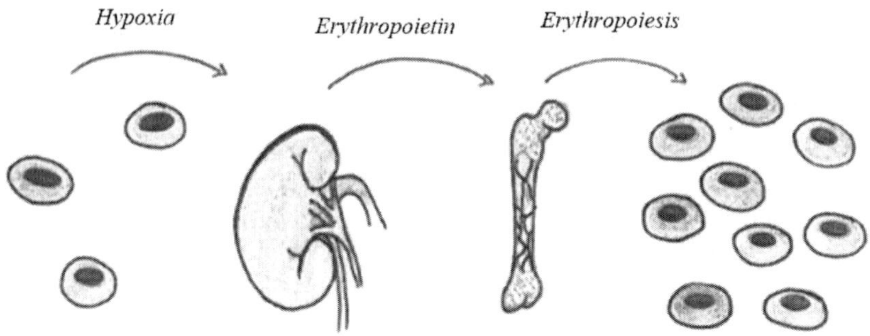

Figure 1. Title: "Activation and Action of Erythropoietin." The figure shows a schematic representation of the action of erythropoietin. The reduced amount of erythrocytes in the blood leads to a decrease in the amount of oxygen in the tissues, which is called hypoxia. Hypoxia is the impetus for the increased secretion of erythropoietin from the kidneys. The released hormone, acting on the bone marrow, stimulates erythropoiesis, which results in an increase in the number of red blood cells, more efficient oxygen transport to tissues and the cessation of hypoxia Source: [Own elaboration].

Erythropoietin plays an important role in the human body, it takes part in hematopoietic processes, stimulating erythropoiesis in hypoxic states. By increasing the number of erythrocytes, it has been used in medicine, primarily in the treatment of anemia, some cancers, kidney and bone marrow diseases and anemia. In the pharmaceutical industry, for therapeutic purposes, recombinant human erythropoietin is used as a drug that stimulates the production of red blood cells in the bone marrow. It should be emphasized that the uncontrolled use of the hormone may lead to a life-threatening condition, therefore its dosage should be supervised by doctors and controlled with blood tests. Testing the level of erythropoietin is used to select the therapy in anemia and in the case of kidney diseases. The analysis of the results allows you to control the effectiveness of the implemented treatment, for example in the treatment of certain types of cancer. Monitoring the level of erythropoietin is also used in doping control among athletes. Carried out to break out the illegal use of doping substances.

Erythropoietin levels are measured from a venous blood sample, usually drawn from a vein in the arm. Before the examination, the patient should not exercise intensively, eat sweet food and drink. It is advisable to collect blood on an empty stomach in the morning, due to the differences in Epo levels during the day (in the morning its level is lower than at night).

References

Bhoopalan SV, Huang LJ, Weiss MJ. Erythropoietin regulation of red blood cell production: from bench to bedside and back. *F1000Res.* 2020 Sep 18;9:F1000 Faculty Rev-1153.

Ehrenreich H, Neubauer AP, Miskowiak K. Erythropoietin in Preterm Infants. *N. Engl. J. Med.* 2020 May 7;382(19):1862.

Juul SE, Comstock BA, Wadhawan R, Mayock DE, Courtney SE, Robinson T, Ahmad KA, Bendel-Stenzel E, Baserga M, LaGamma EF, Downey LC, Rao R, Fahim N, Lampland A, Frantz Iii ID, Khan JY, Weiss M, Gilmore MM, Ohls RK, Srinivasan N, Perez JE, McKay V, Vu PT, Lowe J, Kuban K, O'Shea TM, Hartman AL, Heagerty PJ; PENUT Trial Consortium. A Randomized Trial of Erythropoietin for Neuroprotection in Preterm Infants. *N. Engl. J. Med.* 2020 Jan 16;382(3):233-243.

Sakaguchi Y, Hamano T, Wada A, Masakane I. Types of Erythropoietin - Stimulating Agents and Mortality among Patients Undergoing Hemodialysis. *J. Am. Soc. Nephrol.* 2019 Jun;30(6):1037-1048.

Shih HM, Wu CJ, Lin SL. Physiology and pathophysiology of renal erythropoietin-producing cells. *J. Formos. Med. Assoc.* 2018 Nov;117(11):955-963.

Chapter 15

Glucagon

Bernadetta Jakubowska, Dorota Bartusik-Aebisher*
and David Aebisher
Medical College of The University of Rzeszów, Poland

Abstract

Glucagon plays a very important role, primarily in the control of blood glucose, thus acting in the opposite way to insulin. Only the proper functioning of both hormones is able to ensure and maintain proper and proper homeostasis of the organism's economy, e.g., related to energy expenditure. Glucagon, produced in the alpha cells of the endocrine pancreas, is a key component involved in thermoregulation. Today, interest in glucagon continues to grow. The last fifty years of research conducted by scientists around the world have allowed us to understand both the way glucagon works and its influence and interaction with other hormones in the body. The current research also focuses on the relationship of glucagon with the states of hyperglycemia in diabetes and the anatomical site of glucagon's action with increased energy expenditure.

Keywords: glucagon, insulin, brown adipose tissue (BAT), antidiabetic drugs, gluconeogenesis

The discovery of a hormone acting opposite to the hormone insulin produced by pancreatic beta cells was a landmark event. The existence of glucagon

---

* Corresponding Author's Email: dbartusikaebisher@ur.edu.pl.

In: The Biochemical Guide to Hormones
Editor: David Aebisher
ISBN: 979-8-88697-492-8

reducing blood glucose levels was proved in the 1920s. Pancreatic factors other than insulin have been reported to affect glucose homeostasis in the body. The discovery of glucagon did not end the research era for this protein. Glucagon is a peptide consisting of 29 amino acids and is synthesized in the alpha cells of the pancreas. The GCG gene is responsible for the coding of the glucagon precursor – proglucagon, which is produced by, inter alia, pancreatic alpha cells and L intestinal cells (Hædersdal et al., 2018). Proglucagon is split into the main glucagon and the so-called major fragment of proglucagon. Glucagon is secreted from the pancreatic islets in response to various metabolic signals, such as changes in blood glucose, certain amino acids, and also to stress. Its secretion is influenced by meals containing protein. In addition to the function of lowering blood glucose, glucagon plays an important role, leading to an increased release of amino acids from peripheral organs and, at the same time, to an increase in the oxidation of amino acids in the liver (Hædersdal et al., 2018). It is believed that this hormone also stimulates lipolysis in white adipose tissue, providing energy substrates for organs, including the liver. Glucagon along with adrenaline inhibit glycolysis and stimulate gluconeogenesis in the liver. Recent studies show the complex relationship between glucagon and insulin, not only in the light of antagonists, because the contribution of alpha cells is essential for the proper functioning of pancreatic beta cells (Janah et al., 2019).

One hundred years after the discovery of glucagon, its biological sphere is still not fully understood. Already decades ago, people became interested in the existence of this hormone by conducting research on animals and humans, then the important role of glucagon on the metabolism of amino acids was demonstrated and confirmed. Thanks to modern methods and technologies, knowledge about glucagon is still significantly expanded. We know that glucagon is a polypeptide hormone formed by the alpha cells of the Langerhans islets of the endocrine pancreas. It is made of a precursor composed of 180 amino acids. Glucagon has a biological half-life of 3-6 minutes and is metabolized in the kidneys and liver (Kleinert et al., 2019).

As mentioned earlier, glucagon is a powerful stimulus for the hepatic turnover of amino acids by inducing increased enzyme activity in the urea cycle.

This hormone indirectly regulates several enzymes of the urea cycle at the transcriptional level – this fact is important because the activity of the enzymes determines the ureogenesis capacity. Glucagon activates the transcription of system A amino acid transporters present in the hepatocyte membrane, thus enabling increased amino acid uptake and availability for ureogenesis. It is worth noting that ureogenesis is a substrate-dependent pathway. In view of the above, it is found that glucagon further induces ureogenesis by supplying substrates due to enhanced amino acid uptake (Müller et al., 2017).

Glucagon's ability to increase energy expenditure has been known for over sixty years, but the mechanisms underlying its thermogenic effects remain largely unclear. In recent years, there has been increasing interest in understanding the physiological and cellular underpinnings of glucagon's energy expenditure regulation. This ability was demonstrated initially in rats and then confirmed in humans in 1960. At present, it is still unknown how and in what anatomical locations glucagon acts to increase energy expenditure, or whether various signaling mechanisms are responsible for the acute and chronic thermogenic effects of glucagon (Perry et al., 2020).

In brown adipose tissue (BAT) cells it was noticed in 1966 that glucagon increases oxygen consumption in the above isolated cells, which means that this hormone acts on BAT autonomously, stimulating energy expenditure. The influence of glucagon on energy expenditure is magnified in mice adapted to cold, under experimental conditions in which BAT mass and its ability to produce heat increase. Another study confirmed that administration of glucagon increases blood flow to BAT, which is consistent with the effects of glucagon on vasodilatation and cardiac output. In view of the above, it was found that acute administration of glucagon affects energy expenditure by BAT.

Glucagon, as a counter-regulatory hormone for insulin, plays a key role in maintaining glucose homeostasis, increases hepatic glucose production by increasing glycogenolysis and gluconeogenesis in the liver, and also affects energy expenditure. A thorough understanding of how glucagon and insulin work can facilitate the development of treatments for diseases with impaired production and secretion of these hormones (Perry et al., 2020).

Regulation of the secretion of the above polypeptide hormone has a significant impact on the functioning of the body. Glucagon plays a very important role, primarily in the control of blood glucose, thus acting in the opposite way to insulin. High blood glucose levels inhibit the secretion of glucagon. Only the proper functioning of both hormones is able to ensure and maintain proper and proper homeostasis of the organism's economy, e.g., related to energy expenditure. Glucagon, produced in the alpha cells of the endocrine pancreas, is a key component involved in thermoregulation. The conducted research has proven its physiological and biochemical role in the processes taking place in the cells of brown adipose tissue, glycogenolysis and gluconeogenesis. In addition, it has been proven that it is involved in the hepatic turnover of amino acids. Knowledge about alpha cell dysfunction is useful in the development of new antidiabetic drugs. Today, interest in glucagon continues to grow. The last fifty years of research conducted by scientists around the world have allowed us to understand both the way glucagon works and its influence and interaction with other hormones in the body. These discoveries have led to the development of important drugs for the treatment of abnormal secretions, the way the hormone works. It should be taken into account that the level of knowledge about glucagon is still increasing. The current research also focuses on the relationship of glucagon with the states of hyperglycemia in diabetes and the anatomical site of glucagon's action with increased energy expenditure.

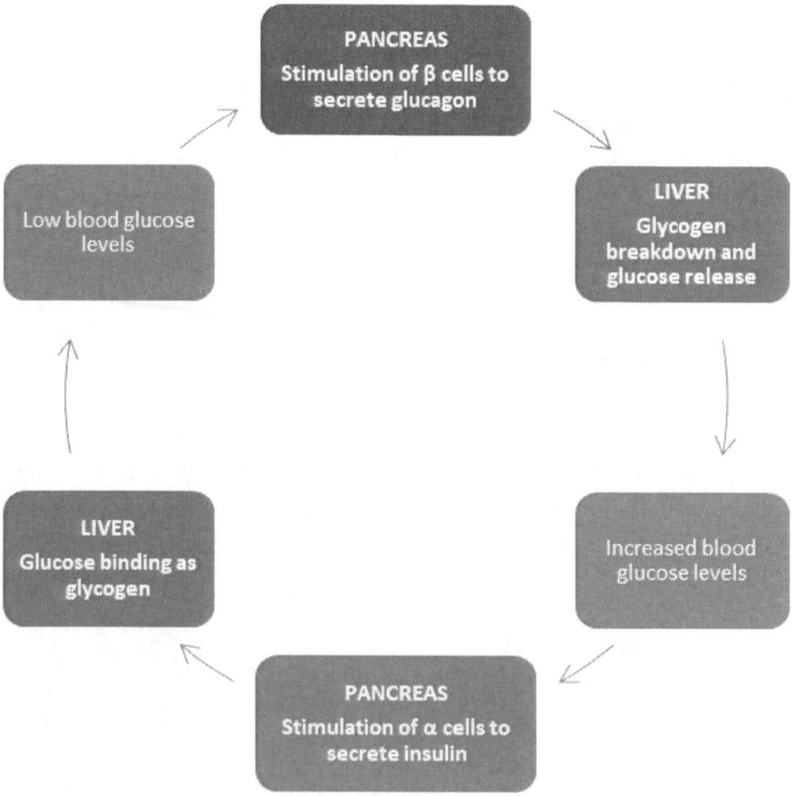

Figure 1. Scheme of the antagonistic effects of glucagon and insulin sensitive to blood glucose levels.

References

Hædersdal S, Lund A, Knop F K, Vilsbøll T. The Role of Glucagon in the Pathophysiology and Treatment of Type 2 Diabetes. *Mayo Clin. Proc.* 2018;93(2):217-239.

Janah L, Kjeldsen S, Galsgaard K D, Winther-Sørensen M, Stojanovska E, Pedersen J, Knop F K, Holst J J, Wewer Albrechtsen N J. Glucagon Receptor Signaling and Glucagon Resistance. *Int. J. Mol. Sci.* 2019;20(13):3314.

Kleinert M, Sachs S, Habegger K M, Hofmann S M, Müller T D. Glucagon Regulation of Energy Expenditure. *Int. J. Mol. Sci.* 2019;20(21):5407.

Müller T D, Finan B, Clemmensen C, DiMarchi R D, Tschöp M H. The New Biology and Pharmacology of Glucagon. *Physiol. Rev.* 2017;97(2):721-766.

Perry R J, Zhang D, Guerra M T, Brill A L, Goedeke L, Nasiri A R, Rabin-Court A, Wang Y, Peng L, Dufour S, Zhang Y, Zhang X M, Butrico G M, Toussaint K, Nozaki Y, Cline G W, Petersen K F, Nathanson M H, Ehrlich B E, Shulman G I. Glucagon stimulates gluconeogenesis by INSP3R1-mediated hepatic lipolysis. *Nature.* 2020; 579(7798): 279-283.

Chapter 16

Estrogen

Julia Trojniak, Dorota Bartusik-Aebisher*
and David Aebisher
Medical College of The University of Rzeszów, Rzeszów, Poland

Abstract

Estrogens – units necessary for the proper functioning of the reproductive system. Estrogens have been widely used in contraceptives. The main risk is the increased likelihood of developing cervical and breast cancer. Estrogens are also used in anti-acne therapies based on hormones. Much less often, but there are estrogen therapies in ovarian dysfunction, e.g., in Turner and Swyer syndromes, premature ovarian failure or in its absence. Hormone replacement therapy (HRT), may also be associated with the treatment of osteoporosis by increasing skeletal weight. They have been shown to reduce ailments such as: depressive symptoms, problems with concentration, insomnia, and problems with appetite. Estrogens are used to improve the cognitive processes of women during the menopause.

Keywords: estrogens, estriol, estrone, stradiol, nuclear-initiated steroid signaling (NISS), membrane-initiated steroid signaling (MISS), Turner syndrome

Estrogens are a group of hormones that are involved, inter alia, in the regulation of the menstrual cycle, determining the second, third and fourth order sexual characteristics in women and conditioning the proper course of

---

* Corresponding Author's Email: dbartusikaebisher@ur.edu.pl.

In: The Biochemical Guide to Hormones
Editor: David Aebisher
ISBN: 979-8-88697-492-8

spermatogenesis in men (their absence determines infertility). Additionally, they control the processes taking place in the epidermis, dermis and all their products. The historical breakthrough in terms of estrogens was 1929, when Adolf Butenandt discovered and described the first of them – estrone. For his research and discovery, in 1939, he was awarded the Nobel Prize (Baker et al. 2017).

Estrogens include:

- estrone (E1);
- estradiol (E2);
- estriol (E3);
- estetrol (E4) - produced during pregnancy.

Apart from naturally occurring estrogens in the organism, there are many chemical compounds with similar activity and functions. This group includes non-steroidal compounds and modifications of physiological estrogens (Baker et al. 2017).

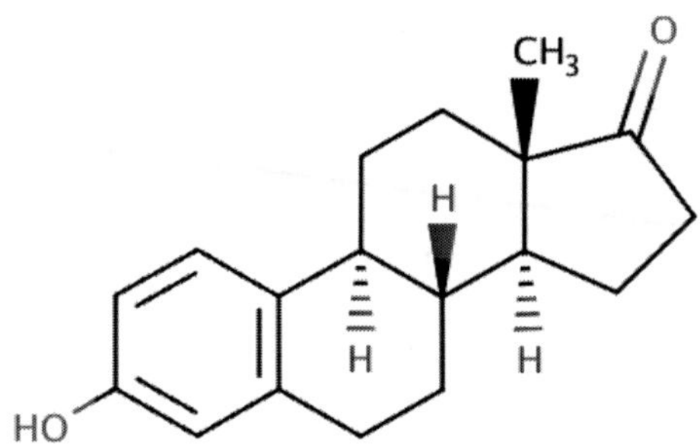

Figure 1. Structural structure of estrone [Own elaboration].

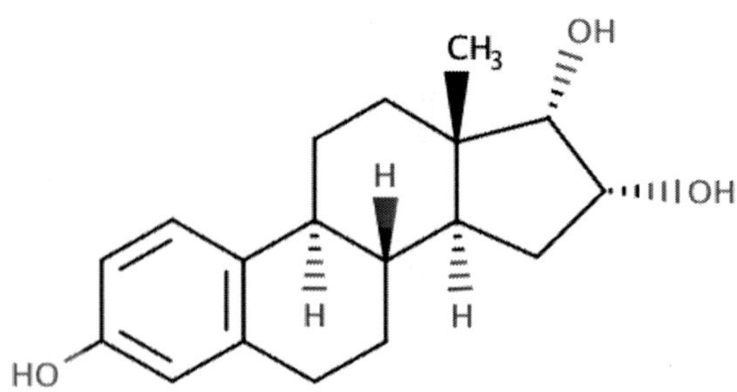

Figure 2. Structural structure of estriol [Own elaboration].

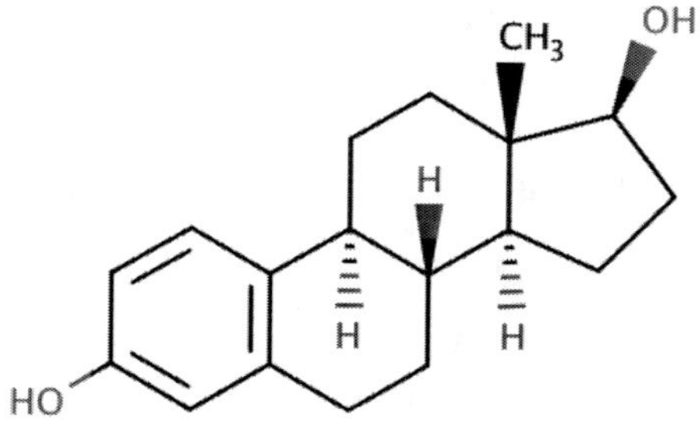

Figure 3. Structural structure of estradiol [Own elaboration].

In women during the activity of the ovaries, estrogen synthesis takes place mainly in granular cells, and after cessation of their activity, this function is temporarily taken over by adipose tissue. In men, synthesis takes place mainly in the Sertoli, Leydig cells, the cells of the drainage tubules and the epididymal duct. Regardless of gender, estrogens are also synthesized and released in the adrenal cortex and the central nervous system – e.g., hippocampus, cerebral cortex and cerebellum (Fuentes et al. 2019).

In terms of their chemical structure, estrogens are classified as steroid hormones. This is due to the presence of a steroid skeleton made of 4 rings in their structure. The phenolic skeleton – the first of these rings – allows a molecule to bind to a receptor. Estrogens differ in their location and number of hydroxyl groups. Due to the fact that these substituents are electron donors, they determine the ability of these hormones to scavenge free radicals. The chemical structure also determines the bioavailability of estrogens. It is related to the rate of first-pass metabolism. The lack of substituents with triple bonds at the 17th carbon atom increases their metabolic rate, which is not inhibited by cytochrome P-450 enzymes (Fuentes et al. 2019).

In estradiol, under the influence of 17-hydroxysteroid dehydrogenase, the hydroxyl group is replaced by the ketone group. The result of these changes is the formation of estrone, with a weaker effect. In the further course of the transformation, also under the influence of 17-hydroxysteroid dehydrogenase and 16-hydroxylase, estriol is formed. During the pathway, intermittent reactions of estrone and estradiol occur, resulting in the formation of hydroxycatechol derivatives, which can then be converted into semiquinones or quinones. Ethinylestradiol is a semi-synthetic estrogen which, due to the presence of triple bonds in its structure, slows down the above-described processes. This results in an increase in its activity, slower elimination from the body, as well as an increase in its half-life (13-27h) (Hewitt et al. 2018).

The most understood functional signaling pathways for estrogens are:

- NISS trail (nuclear-initiated steroid signaling);
- MISS trail (membrane-initiated steroid signaling).

NISS pathway is signaling initiated in the zone of the cell nucleus. Initially, the ligand binds to the receptor, and then the complex is transported to the nucleus. In this structure, receptor dimerization and binding to an element of the estrogen response takes place. This is crucial for the rate of gene transcription as it modifies the late tissue response.

The MISS pathway is signaling initiated in the area of the cell membrane. Estradiol activates membrane binding site and initiates intracellular signaling pathways. As a result, a rapid cellular response is produced (Hess et al. 2018).

There are two types of receptors:

- ERα;
- ERβ.

They are located both in the cell membrane and in the nucleus.

The differentiation of the cellular response to stimulation of estrogen receptors may be due to several reasons, including:

- different affinity of the hormone molecule for the receptor protein;
- ligand multifunctionality – inhibitor or activator, depending on the site of attachment;
- different activity and distribution depending on the target tissues and organs.

The correct level of estrogen is necessary for the proper functioning of the body of both women and men.

Standards for women:

- Estron - in the reproductive period 17-200 ng/l, in the postmenopausal period 7-40 ng/l
- Estradiol - different norms depending on the cycle phase - follicular phase: 30-120 ng/l (110-440 pmol/l), ovulation: 130-370 ng/l (477-1358 pmol/l), luteal phase: 70-250 ng/l (257-917 pmol/l). In the postmenopausal period, the normal level of estradiol is <10 ng/L.
- Estriol - less than 80 ng/l

Standards for men:

- Estron: 10-60 ng/l
- Estradiol: 10-40 ng/L
- Estriol: <160 ng/L

Estrogen deficiency can have a very negative effect on the body, e.g., at a young age it can cause ovarian hypoplasia, Sweyer syndrome, Turner syndrome. In adult women, the effects include premature ovarian failure or postmenopausal transition.

Too much estrogen is known as hyperestrogenism. In women, it manifests itself as a disturbance of the menstrual cycle. This may be due to, for example, ovarian cancer, stress, poor diet or genetics. Complications may include blood clots, blockages, edema and cholelithiasis (Wilkinson et al. 2017).

Estrogens have been widely used in contraceptives. Due to the wide range of side effects, the aim is to reduce their concentration in the drug. The main risk is the increased likelihood of developing cervical and breast cancer. It is worth mentioning, however, that the probability of developing ovarian cancer during the treatment decreases. Estrogens are also used in anti-acne therapies based on hormones. Much less often, but there are estrogen therapies in ovarian dysfunction, e.g., in Turner and Swyer syndromes, premature ovarian failure or in its absence.

These hormones are increasingly used in replacement therapy (HRT), where low levels of these substances help to eliminate many of the symptoms of menopause. Hormone replacement therapy may also be associated with the treatment of osteoporosis by increasing skeletal weight.

Estrogens are also used to improve the cognitive processes of women during the menopause. They have been shown to reduce ailments such as: depressive symptoms, problems with concentration, insomnia, and problems with appetite (Wilkinson et al. 2017).

References

Baker JM, Al-Nakkash L, Herbst-Kralovetz MM. Estrogen-gut microbiome axis: Physiological and clinical implications. *Maturitas*. 2017;103:45-53.

Fuentes N, Silveyra P. Estrogen receptor signaling mechanisms. *Adv. Protein Chem. Struct. Biol*. 2019;116:135-170.

Hess RA, Cooke PS. Estrogen in the male: a historical perspective. *Biol. Reprod.* 2018;99(1):27-44.

Hewitt SC, Korach KS. Estrogen Receptors: New Directions in the New Millennium. *Endocr. Rev.* 2018;39(5):664-675.

Wilkinson HN, Hardman MJ. The role of estrogen in cutaneous ageing and repair. *Maturitas.* 2017;103:60-64.

Chapter 17

Insulin

Gabriela Barszcz, Dorota Bartusik-Aebisher*
and David Aebisher
Medical College of The University of Rzeszów, Poland

Abstract

Insulin, as an anabolic hormone, plays a key role in the metabolism of carbohydrates. Its reference values are 2.6 - 24.9 μU / ml. The action and stimulation of this hormone is extremely complex and depends on mechanisms originating in many organs. By circulating in the blood, insulin enables the cells to absorb glucose, which lowers blood sugar levels in the bloodstream. The very examination of the insulin level allows to assess the diagnosis of the condition of the endocrine and digestive systems, as well as the general functioning and efficiency of the body. In addition, insulin, getting to the muscles and adipose tissue, supports glucose uptake by contractile fibers and fat cells.

Keywords: insulin, LXR, USF1, receptor, amino acids, hormone

The discovery of insulin in 1922 by Frederick Banting and his assistants Charles Best, James Collip and John Macleod was one of the most important, as it was a breakthrough in the treatment of diabetes. Insulin is a peptide hormone with an anabolic effect. It plays a vital role in the body by stimulating the metabolism of carbohydrates, lipids and proteins. In addition, it stimulates the absorption of glucose from the blood into adipose tissue and skeletal muscles, and stores it in the form of glycogen when there is an excess of it in

* Corresponding Author's Email: dbartusikaebisher@ur.edu.pl.

In: The Biochemical Guide to Hormones
Editor: David Aebisher
ISBN: 979-8-88697-492-8

the blood. It also controls glucose consumption in target cells, DNA replication as well as protein synthesis (Cernea et al., 2020).

Insulin is produced by the beta cells (β) of the islets of the pancreas (Langerhans), which also owes it its name – Latin. "Insula" means an island. Inside these cells, glucose undergoes modifications in the Krebs cycle, leading to the formation of ATP, which regulates the ion current within the islands and the release of the contents – which confirms that the most important stimulus for insulin production is glucose (Cernea et al., 2020).

Insulin secreted by the pancreas controls gluconeogenesis, muscle and liver glycolysis, adipogenesis and adipocyte lysis of adipose tissue, e.g., in the case of excess energy substrates, it inhibits gluconeogenesis and glucogenolysis. It also has a wide range of action – it reaches almost all tissues of the body. After attaching to a specific receptor – IR – it activates a tyrosine kinase that activates proteins from the IRS family, and further the induction of specific metabolic pathways, such as the synthesis of cholesterol or fatty acids (Moussavi et al., 2019).

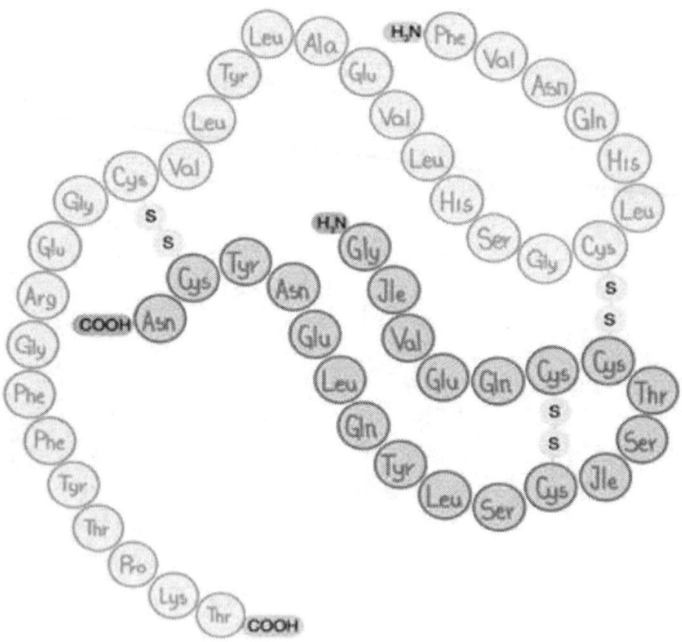

Figure 1. Schematic structure of insulin taking into account the sequence of amino acids in the A chain (blue) and in the B chain (orange), and the places of disulfide bridges.

The human insulin molecule consists of two polypeptide chains – A (21 amino acids) and B (30 amino acids), which are connected with each other by disulfide bridges, but the entire molecule contains 3 disulfide bridges – one contained in the A chain, and two chains connecting A and B chains.

Insulin as an anabolic hormone is responsible for many important mechanisms functioning in the human body. The most important function is to control blood glucose levels. Incorrect production of it may lead to serious disorders, such as type 2 diabetes – in this case, increasing insulin resistance is directly related to the disturbance of insulin secretion from pancreatic cells, but the underlying disease may also include pathology of intestinal hormone secretion, affecting insulin secretion, not associated with an increase in blood glucose (Pérez et al., 2020). Even without the stimulus, insulin secretion is constant, but at a low level. We also observe changes in the intensity of insulin secretion depending on the time of day – the highest in the morning, and weaker in the evening. The human body requires approximately 50 units of insulin per day to function properly.

In response to an excess of circulating glucose in the blood (hyperglycemia), preproinsulin is formed on the ribosomes of the rough endoplasmic reticulum of the beta cells of Langerhans islets, which consists of proinsulin, composed of 84 amino acids (including the B chain – 30 amino acids, a 33-amino acid C-linker peptide) and the 21 amino acid chain of A) and the 23 amino acid signal peptide. Proinsulin, or "high insulin," is inactive in the body, and it is difficult to distinguish it from the insulin molecule. Only small amounts of it enter the circulatory system. After the formation of disulfide bonds between the A and B chains, pro-insulin goes to the Golgi apparatus, where after about 1 hour, it becomes its active form – insulin. The endopeptidases contained therein help to remove the C chain. The half-life of insulin in the circulation is 5 minutes (Selivanova et al., 2018).

Glucose, via the transporter GLUT 2, penetrates into the beta cells of the Langerhans islets. An increase in its concentration in the blood increases the production of ATP, which by blocking potassium channels leads to depolarization of the cell membrane. Progressive depolarization increases the intracellular current of calcium ions as the membrane permeability to them increases - this in turn affects the secretion of insulin outside the membrane. Insulin exocytosis is also influenced by: amino acids, free fatty acids, ketone bodies, glucagon, secretin, and sulfonylurea drugs. On the other hand, the blocking of insulin secretion is caused by adrenaline and noradrenaline. The way insulin reduces glucose is transported to adipose tissue or muscles via the

GLUT 4 transporter. It also stimulates the liver to store glucose in the form of glycogen (Selivanova et al., 2018).

Insulin blocks the release of free fatty acids from adipose tissue, which reduces their concentration in the blood. By enhancing lipogenesis and causing a cascade of other activities, it increases the uptake of glucose - depending on its concentration - by adipose tissue with the help of GLUT 4. Indirectly, it also increases the synthesis of fatty acids and acylglycerols.

Human insulin has a molecular weight of 5734, but under various conditions, it can take the form of various polymers, the molecular weight of which is between 12,000 - 48,000. Metabolic activity is determined by the disulfide bridges between the A and B chains, which give it an appropriate structure. Changes within the chain or between them lead to the inactivation of this protein (Sharma et al., 2019).

The released insulin acts on its specific receptors, present in the membranes of cells of almost all tissues - IR with tyrosine kinase activity, activating proteins from the IRS family. Due to the activation of these proteins, the appropriate impulse conduction pathways can be stimulated. Among these important receptor proteins, PI3K plays a significant role, which, through the reaction cascade, contributes to the enhancement of glycogen synthesis, induction of protein synthesis and cell survival. Among the IRS receptors, there are also those that regulate SREB1 and SREB2, i.e., transcription factors that trigger the synthesis of fatty acids and cholesterol. Activation of LXR and USF1 receptors by insulin contributes to the synthesis of free fatty acids (Sharma et al., 2019).

Insulin, as an anabolic hormone, plays a key role in the metabolism of carbohydrates. Its reference values are 2.6 - 24.9 μU / ml. The action and stimulation of this hormone is extremely complex and depends on mechanisms originating in many organs. The most important organ is the pancreas, whose beta cells produce and export insulin in response to a stimulus such as glucose concentration. By circulating in the blood, insulin enables the cells to absorb glucose, which lowers blood sugar levels in the bloodstream. Although insulin is mainly involved in controlling blood sugar levels, it is also involved in the metabolism of fats and proteins. It is a key hormone for the health of every human being, as abnormalities resulting from its disturbed levels can result in serious diseases - very high glucose levels, or hyperglycemia, can even lead to death as a result of a diabetic coma, if the condition is not treated. This condition occurs in patients with diabetes, which is directly related to the disturbance of insulin secretion. The very examination of the insulin level allows to assess the diagnosis of the condition of the endocrine and digestive systems, as well as the general functioning and efficiency of the body. In addition, insulin, getting to the muscles and adipose tissue, supports glucose uptake by contractile fibers and fat cells. The excess insulin remains degraded in the kidneys, where the hormone stops working and the body's metabolic balance is maintained.

References

Cernea S, Raz I. Insulin Therapy: Future Perspectives. *Am. J. Ther.* 2020 Jan/Feb;27 (1):e121-e132.

Moussavi K, Fitter S, Gabrielson S W, Koyfman A, Long B. Management of Hyperkalemia With Insulin and Glucose: Pearls for the Emergency Clinician. *J. Emerg. Med.* 2019 Jul;57(1):36-42.

Pérez A, Ramos A, Carreras G. Insulin Therapy in Hospitalized Patients. *Am. J. Ther.* 2020 Jan/Feb;27(1):e71-e78.

Selivanova O M, Grishin S Y, Glyakina A V, Sadgyan A S, Ushakova N I, Galzitskaya O V. Analysis of Insulin Analogs and the Strategy of Their Further Development. *Biochemistry (Mosc).* 2018 Jan;83(Suppl 1):S146-S162.

Sharma A K, Taneja G, Kumar A, Sahu M, Sharma G, Kumar A, Sardana S, Deep A. Insulin analogs: Glimpse on contemporary facts and future prospective. *Life Sci.* 2019 Feb 15;219:90-99.

Chapter 18

Parathyroid Hormone (PTH)

**Łukasz Łukasiewicz, Dorota Bartusik-Aebisher*
and David Aebisher**
Medical College of The University of Rzeszów, Poland

Abstract

Parathyroid hormone (PTH) is the major secretion product of the parathyroid glands. In the human body, it is mainly responsible for the hormonal regulation of the balance of two extremely important elements – calcium and phosphate. PTH has found clinical application as a replacement therapy for hypoparathyroidism. In diagnostics, its concentration level in the blood allows the evaluation of the work of the parathyroid glands. The regulation of PTH levels in the blood is closely related to the concentration of extracellular calcium. The mechanism responsible for this control is a negative feedback mediated by the calcium-sensing receptor (CaSR). PTH may also play a physiological role in enhancing bone formation, especially in spongy and to some extent in the cortex of the bone. This action has been used in the treatment of anabolic osteoporosis.

Keywords: fibroblast, parathyroid hormone, biosynthesis, cells, hyperparathyroidism, vitamin D

Parathyroid hormone is a polypeptide hormone consisting of 84 amino acids. In the human body, it is mainly responsible for the hormonal regulation of the

---

* Corresponding Author's Email dbartusikaebisher@ur.edu.pl.

In: The Biochemical Guide to Hormones
Editor: David Aebisher
ISBN: 979-8-88697-492-8

balance of two extremely important elements - calcium and phosphate. In diagnostics, its concentration level in the blood allows the evaluation of the work of the parathyroid glands.

The main cells of the parathyroid gland are responsible for the production of PTH. A characteristic phenomenon is that PTH is constantly produced by cells, stored in granules and secreted under certain conditions. The release of parathyroid hormone depends on the level of calcium, phosphate and vitamin D3 metabolite in the blood serum. Once released, it is an important hormone that affects the health of our bones. Laboratory standards differ from each other for various reasons, i.e., the method of determination and the material collected for testing, but we can accept 10-60 pg / ml. The test is usually ordered when there are symptoms that may indicate an overactive or underactive parathyroid gland (Goltzman et al., 2018).

Hyperparathyroidism is a common endocrinopathy, caused by the uncontrolled growth of parathyroid cells. Hypercalcaemia develops in post-hypertension as a result of the excessive automatic secretion of PTH. Secondary hyperparathyroidism is a common complication of chronic renal failure, which results in significant glandular hyperplasia, especially in patients undergoing frequent dialysis. As a natural substance that affects bone health, it has been used in the treatment of postmenopausal women and men with hypogonadism struggling with osteoporosis (Goltzman et al., 2018).

The initial product, which is encoded by the mRNA, is the pre-proparathormone (PreProPTH), consisting of 115 amino acids. During the first proteolytic cleavage, 25 amino acids are cleaved from the N-terminal side. This process produces proparathormone (ProPTH). In the Golgi, ProPTH loses a further six amino acids, resulting in the formation of eighty-four amino acid parathyroid hormone. It is accumulated in the granules of the main cells of the parathyroid glands (Leder et al., 2017).

The regulation of PTH levels in the blood is closely related to the concentration of extracellular calcium. The mechanism responsible for this control is a negative feedback mediated by the calcium-sensing receptor (CaSR). CaSR is one of the receptors associated with the G protein, which responds to extracellular changes in calcium levels. A decrease in serum ionized calcium (< 0.98mmol / L) stimulates PTH secretion, while an increase (> 1.13mmol / L) inhibits PTH release and stimulates calcitonin secretion. Increasing the concentration of extracellular calcium causes a conformational change of the CaSR receptor, and in turn initiates the intracellular path of phospholipase C. The effect of DAG and IP3 is an increased concentration of intracellular calcium, inhibition of vesicle fusion and parathyroid hormone exocytosis. A second mechanism that regulates PTH secretion involves fibroblast growth factor 23 (Leun et al., 2021).

Fibroblast growth factor 23 is an element of the FGF23-bone-kidney axis, which in the light of recent studies should be considered a new regulatory system, playing a role comparable to the PTH-vitamin D axis. The place of synthesis are osteoblasts and osteocytes, therefore bone tissue is considered an organ internal secretion responsible for the regulation of calcium and phosphate metabolism. FGF23 targets the kidneys by inhibiting phosphate reabsorption in the proximal tubules, reducing the synthesis of 1,25 (OH)2D and the expression of the Klotho protein (FGF23 cofactor). (Witkowska-Sędek). With the correct concentration of calcium, PTH determines the processes of bone remodeling, i.e., stimulates their remodeling (resorption and neoplastic processes). During hypocalcemia, the secretion of parathyroid hormone in the blood increases and the concentration of the active form of vitamin D3 increases, which acts permissively, i.e., enhances the effect of parathyroid hormone (Wojda et al., 2018).

The effect of parathyroid hormone on the kidneys consists in inhibiting the reabsorption of phosphates in the proximal tubules and increasing their excretion in the urine, while increasing the reabsorption of Ca2+ ions in the distal tubules and reducing their excretion in the urine. Parathyroid hormone plays a very important role in controlling the production of the hormonal form of vitamin D3 in the kidneys by stimulating the activity of the enzyme hydroxylase responsible for the formation of the active form 1,25(OH)2D3 from the 25(OH) D3 precursor. The absorption of calcium from the gastrointestinal tract is not without the influence of PTH, it is enhanced mainly by the active form of vitamin D3 (Wojda et al., 2018).

Parathyroid hormone (PTH) is the major secretion product of the parathyroid glands. In states of hypocalcemia, it causes an increase in calcium reabsorption by the kidneys, stimulates the production of active vitamin D in the kidneys, which ultimately leads to an increase in intestinal calcium absorption and mobilizes calcium stored in the bones in the form of hydroxyapatite by increasing the turnover. Therefore, PTH has found clinical application as a replacement therapy for hypoparathyroidism. PTH may also play a physiological role in enhancing bone formation, especially in spongy and to some extent in the cortex of the bone. This action has been used in the treatment of anabolic osteoporosis.

References

Goltzman D, Mannstadt M, Marcocci C. Physiology of the Calcium-Parathyroid Hormone-Vitamin D Axis. *Front Horm. Res.* 2018; 50: 1-13.

Goltzman D. Physiology of Parathyroid Hormone. *Endocrinol. Metab Clin. North Am.* 2018; 47(4): 743-758.

Leder BZ. Parathyroid Hormone and Parathyroid Hormone-Related Protein Analogs in Osteoporosis Therapy. *Curr. Osteoporos. Rep.* 2017; 15(2): 110-119.

Leun EKY. Parathyroid hormone. *Adv. Clin. Chem.* 2021; 101: 41-93.

Wojda SJ, Donahue SW. Parathyroid hormone for bone regeneration. *J. Orthop. Res.* 2018; 36(10): 2586-2594.

Chapter 19

Progesterone

**Klaudia Kusz, Dorota Bartusik-Aebisher*
and David Aebisher**
Medical College of The University of Rzeszów, Rzeszów, Poland

Abstract

Progesterone is a unique, endogenous hormone that can be secreted by the corpus luteum and placenta, but also synthesized in the CNS and PSN. It works with estrogen, thanks to which it regulates the monthly cycle and inhibits the resorption of calcium from the bones, preventing the occurrence of diseases such as osteoporosis. The unbalanced level may adversely affect the cycle in women, as well as health, leading to, for example, thromboembolic diseases. Current scientific discoveries prove that progesterone is not only useful in the functioning of the human reproductive system, but can also play a significant role in its clinical application. It creates a range of possibilities in hormone therapies. It has a potential role in clinical situations during the treatment of, for example, TBI, Alzheimer's disease or prostate enlargement.

Keywords: progesterone, hormone, hyperprolactinemia, neurosteroids, hypothyroidism, chronic obstructive pulmonary disease (COPD)

Progesterone is an endogenous hormone belonging to the group of steroid hormones – more precisely to progestogens. The progesterone molecule is a derivative of cholesterol. It is often called the "pregnancy hormone" or

---

* Corresponding Author's Email: dbartusikaebisher@ur.edu.pl.

In: The Biochemical Guide to Hormones
Editor: David Aebisher
ISBN: 979-8-88697-492-8

"pregnancy care giver." It is secreted from the cortex of the adrenal gland and in the ovary by the corpus luteum in response to the stimulating effects of luteinizing hormone during the second half of the menstrual cycle and during the first ten weeks of pregnancy. Later, the placenta is also responsible for its production. It also plays a very important role in maintaining the early stages of pregnancy. It enables the endometrium to pass from the proliferative to the secretory phase, causes gradual growth of the uterine muscle and stimulates its mucosa to secrete nutrients (Pickar et al., 2018). During the menstrual cycle, it causes the growth of capillaries due to increased vascularization and blood flow. A fall in progesterone levels at the right time in the cycle causes the flaking lining of the womb to shed and causes menstruation, but it can also be a symptom of a miscarriage. The discussed hormone, however, does not only affect the female reproductive system. Its functions also include stimulating the respiratory center, which allows it to cover the increased demand for oxygen. It also affects the thermoregulation center in the hypothalamus, which causes an increase in body temperature. Progesterone stimulates the development of the mammary glands by influencing the glandular alveoli and the epithelium of the exit ducts. In this case, this hormone "cooperates" with estrogen, which increases the number of progesterone receptors. The "pregnancy hormone" has been widely used in hormone therapies, e.g., in the case of miscarriages or premature births, as well as in hormonal contraception (Pickar et al., 2018).

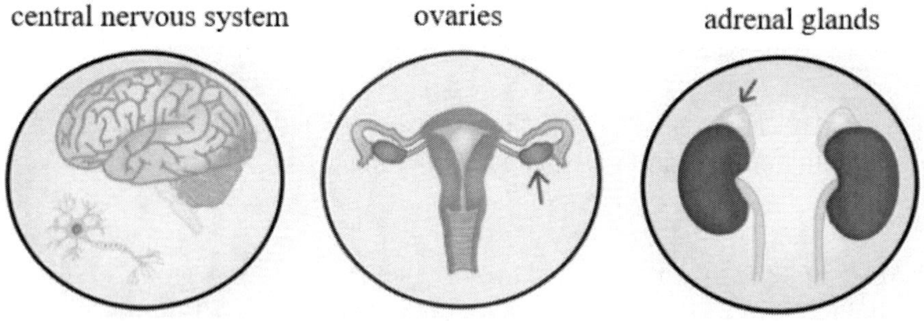

Figure 1. Progesterone synthesis sites [Own elaboration].

Progesterone and other progestins have little effect on bones. Progestin receptors have been identified on osteoclasts and osteoblasts, leading to the hypothesis that it inhibits bone resorption by stimulating calcitonin secretion, as is the case with estrogen. Progesterone alone, however, has very little effect, however, the combination of MPA and estradiol induce a significant decline in osteoporotic cells, which is effective in preventing osteoporosis.

Progesterone has been classified as neurosteroids – hormones that are synthesized from cholesterol in the central and peripheral nervous systems. Regardless of its origin, progesterone has been shown to have neuroprotective and neurotrophic effects. This hormone is very important in the regeneration of the CNS and PSN, as well as in the production of myelin and remyelination. In addition, progesterone, after conversion to allopregnanolone, and by affecting GABA A receptors, causes anxiolytic, anticonvulsant and sedative effects. The negative effect of lowering the level of progesterone on the occurrence of the premenstrual syndrome manifested by aggressive behavior and fatigue, which is caused by the deficiency of progesterone in this phase of the cycle, has also been proven (Henderson et al., 2018).

Progesterone is useful for identifying clinical complications and making diagnoses. It is also often combined with estrogen, which is used as a contraceptive. It is used to treat amenorrhea, anovulation and endometrial hyperplasia. It is also given to women during dysfunctional vaginal bleeding, which occurs especially during puberty and in postmenopausal women. In addition to reproductive uses, progesterone is used by clinicians to treat high blood pressure and chronic obstructive pulmonary disease (COPD) (Jewson et al., 2020).

In men, progesterone is produced by the testes and the adrenal cortex. It influences the process of sperm capacitation, facilitating it, thanks to which an acrosomal reaction involving the penetration of the sperm into the oocyte is possible. It also protects against prostate cancer by inhibiting the conversion of testosterone into dihydrotestosterone. Typically, however, this hormone in the case of the male sex is considered a physiologically insignificant by-product in steroidogenesis, and its secretion and receptor function are the result of the action of estrogens (Coomarasamy et al., 2020).

Progesterone plays the most important role in childbearing age, and if the body does not produce enough of it, it can lead to problems with getting or maintaining a pregnancy. It can also cause irregular or complete cessation of monthly cycles. It also leads to frequent mood swings, depression, hot flashes, headaches, night sweats, weight gain and vaginal dryness. The deficiency of this hormone may be caused, inter alia, by low cholesterol, which is its precursor. Hypothyroidism is another cause of progesterone deficiency as the thyroid gland cannot produce enough of the hormones T3 and T4 to regulate the entire endocrine system. Chronic stress causes the production of large amounts of cortisol, which hinders the production of progesterone –

compounds used to produce progesterone. A condition caused by the increased production of the hormone prolactin by the pituitary gland – hyperprolactinemia has a negative effect on the production of sex hormone precursors, including the reduction of progesterone synthesis. High progesterone levels are characterized by swelling, water retention, slower blood flow, and varicose veins. In the case of men, there are also diseases such as gynecomastia, erectile dysfunction and oligospermia – a reduced amount of sperm in semen. Its excess may be caused by the presence of a multiple pregnancy. It also proves the possibility of cysts on the ovaries, disorders of the adrenal glands and ovarian cancer (Trabert et al., 2020).

Progesterone is therefore a unique, endogenous hormone that can be secreted by the corpus luteum and placenta, but also synthesized in the CNS and PSN. It is necessary for the proper course of pregnancy and its maintenance. It works with estrogen, thanks to which it regulates the monthly cycle and inhibits the resorption of calcium from the bones, preventing the occurrence of diseases such as osteoporosis. It is a neurosteroid that has a very positive effect on the nervous system and is responsible for its regeneration and the production of myelin sheaths. It can protect against brain damage through a number of mechanisms. Nevertheless, its unbalanced level may adversely affect the cycle in women, as well as health, leading to, for example, thromboembolic diseases.

Current scientific discoveries prove that progesterone is not only useful in the functioning of the human reproductive system, but can also play a significant role in its clinical application. It creates a range of possibilities in hormone therapies. It has a potential role in clinical situations during the treatment of, for example, TBI, Alzheimer's disease or prostate enlargement.

This hormone still arouses great scientific interest and engages researchers from many fields – biochemistry, gynecology and obstetrics, pharmacology, and endocrinology. Continuously progressing research may contribute to a better understanding and understanding of its impact on the body, thanks to which it will be possible to obtain a more complete knowledge about its safety and effectiveness, and therefore to its more effective use in various fields – medical and scientific.

References

Coomarasamy A, Devall A J, Brosens J J, Quenby S, Stephenson M D, Sierra S, Christiansen O B, Small R, Brewin J, Roberts T E, Dhillon-Smith R, Harb H, Noordali

H, Papadopoulou A, Eapen A, Prior M, Di Renzo G C, Hinshaw K, Mol B W, Lumsden M A, Khalaf Y, Shennan A, Goddijn M, van Wely M, Al-Memar M, Bennett P, Bourne T, Rai R, Regan L, Gallos I D. Micronized vaginal progesterone to prevent miscarriage: a critical evaluation of randomized evidence. *Am. J. Obstet. Gynecol.* 2020; 223(2): 167-176.

Henderson V W. Progesterone and human cognition. *Climacteric*. 2018; 21(4): 333-340.

Jewson M, Purohit P, Lumsden M A. Progesterone and abnormal uterine bleeding/menstrual disorders. *Best Pract. Res. Clin. Obstet. Gynaecol*. 2020; 69: 62-73.

Pickar J H. Progesterone. *Climacteric*. 2018; 21(4): 305.

Trabert B, Sherman M E, Kannan N, Stanczyk FZ. Progesterone and Breast Cancer. *Endocr. Rev.* 2020; 41(2): 320–44.

Chapter 20

Norepinephrine

Olga Pastuszko, Dorota Bartusik-Aebisher*
and David Aebisher
Medical College of The University of Rzeszów, Rzeszów, Poland

Abstract

Norepinephrine is known as norepinephrine. Norepinephrine is a neurohormone and neurotransmitter, acts on many receptors, reducing cortical activity, either limiting the outflow of neurotransmitters, or increasing sensitivity to inhibitory signaling. It is one of the most important neurotransmitters in the sympathetic nervous system. It plays a key role in all forebrain functions, such as perception, memory, learning and homeostasis, and its dysfunction is closely related to both neurodegenerative diseases and central nervous system disorders. Norepinephrine stimulates both α- and β-adrenergic receptors. The activated β receptors increase the contractility and excitability of the heart, and accelerate its action. In wakefulness, the concentration increases, and much higher levels are observed in states of stress and danger.

Keywords: norepinephrine, adrenoceptors, hyperpolarised cyclic nucleotide-gated (HCN), vesicles

Norepinephrine is otherwise known as norepinephrine – this term is more common, heard more often. The word norepinephrine comes from the Latin

* Corresponding Author's Email: dbartusikaebisher@ur.edu.pl.

In: The Biochemical Guide to Hormones
Editor: David Aebisher
ISBN: 979-8-88697-492-8

term which can be translated as "around the kidneys." Norepinephrine is an organic chemical compound belonging to catecholamines, a derivative of the amino acid – tyrosine. It is one of the most important neurotransmitters in the sympathetic nervous system. Under physiological conditions, it is formed in postganglionic adrenergic neurons and pheochromocytomas of the adrenal medulla. Almost all of the brain's noradrenergic fibers are formed in the nuclei of the brainstem labeled A1-A7 (about half of the neurons belong to the nucleus of the brainstem, the bluish site) (Brown et al., 2020).

Norepinephrine has many effects and mediates a number of functions in living organisms. It plays a key role in all forebrain functions, such as perception, memory, learning and homeostasis, and its dysfunction is closely related to both neurodegenerative diseases and central nervous system disorders. The effects of norepinephrine are mediated by two separate superfamilies of receptors, called alpha and beta adrenergic receptors. They are further broken down into subgroups that have specific roles in modulating behavior and cognition. Adrenoceptors are located on the periphery and in the CNS, and selective alpha and beta receptor agonists and antagonists are used to assess their function. Its lowest concentration in the human body is observed during sleep. In wakefulness, the concentration increases, and much higher levels are observed in states of stress and danger (Brown et al., 2020).

Norepinephrine, catecholamine, is derived from l-tyrosine, an aromatic amino acid found in body fluids and absorbed by cells that produce norepinephrine.

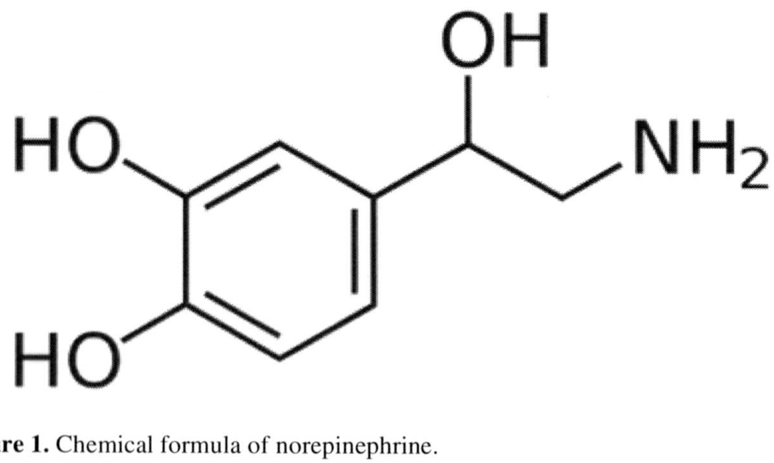

Figure 1. Chemical formula of norepinephrine.

Through various intermediate steps (Figure 2), L-tyrosine is converted into norepinephrine and finally into its methylated form, epinephrine, in cells containing phenylethanolamine N-methyltransferase. The first cytosolic enzyme, tyrosine hydroxylase, is inhibited by overproduction of norepinephrine and is the rate-limiting step in the regulation of norepinephrine synthesis. Tyrosine hydroxylase is found only in the cytosol in catecholamine-containing cells and is used as a marker for the detection of adrenergic neurons. Dopamine β-hydroxylase is also used as a selectable marker for catecholamine-containing cells, but is localized in secretory vesicles, usually associated with the membrane; however, a small amount is soluble and released with the vesicle content following exocytosis (Kohno et al., 2019).

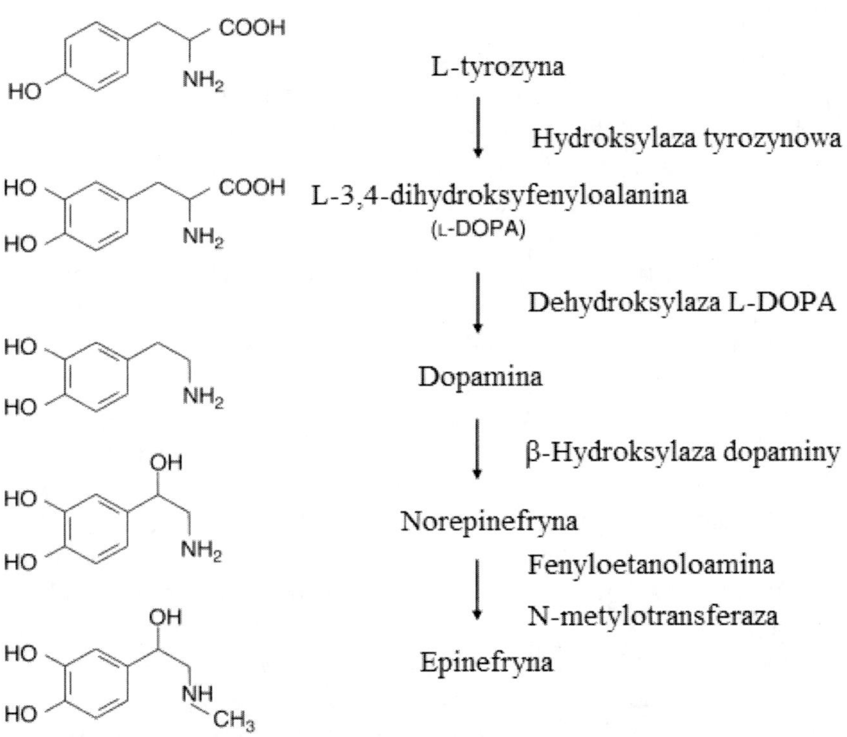

Figure 2. The process of norepinephrine biosynthesis from L-tyrosine.

Norepinephrine is stored in vesicles (also called storage granules) in nerve endings that concentrate it and protect it from metabolism until it is released after nerve stimulation. The main mechanism by which the action of norepinephrine is terminated is the reuptake back into the nerve end by a high affinity transporter. Norepinephrine can also be metabolized to inactive products. Inhibition of any of these processes increases the synaptic level of norepinephrine and prolongs its action. Norepinephrine is metabolized by the enzymes monoamine oxidase and catechol-O-methyltransferase to 3-methoxy-4-hydroxymandelic acid and 3-methoxy-4-hydroxyphenylglycol (MHPG). The major blood and urine metabolite is MHPG, and levels of this metabolite are often used to assess the functional status of the noradrenergic system in humans (Sicherer et al., 2017).

The signaling of norepinephrine in cortical neurons is highly variable, possibly affecting all neuron populations. A major consequence of norepinephrine signaling, which is common with other neuromodulators, is its ability to limit the pulse frequency adaptation of cortical neurons. Norepinephrine, by activating β-adrenergic receptors, facilitates the transmission of action potential trains by suppressing $Ca2^{+}$ activated K^{+} (SK) channels and hyperpolarization conductivity (IADH) in the cAMP and PKA dependent pathway. Additionally, emotional stress and nonselective activation of β-adrenergic receptors have a profound effect on synaptic strength by increasing the postsynaptic insertion of α-amino-3-hydroxy-5-methyl-4-isoxazolpropionic acid (AMPA). Furthermore, in the prefrontal cortex, norepinephrine activates α2-adrenergic receptors and closes hyperpolarised cyclic nucleotide-gated (HCN) channels, a non-selective cation channel, by lowering intracellular cAMP levels. The closure of HCN channels lowers the threshold of action potential generation in spatially-tuned prefrontal cortex neurons related to delay, resulting in increased network connectivity related to spatial working memory. In summary, the increased excitatory effect of norepinephrine is mainly due to its modulation of SK and HCN channels with a concomitant increase in AMPA receptor trafficking (Sicherer et al., 2017).

However, norepinephrine also plays a role in reducing excitatory transmission. Activation of α2-adrenergic receptors reduces the influx of calcium ($Ca2^{+}$) through voltage-gated $Ca2^{+}$ channels (Cav2.2, N-type calcium channels) and reduces the release of neurotransmitters. This effect is mediated by the βγ G protein subunit and is independent of intracellular cAMP concentrations. Activation of the α1-adrenergic receptors, however, may prevent inhibition of the Cav2.2 α2-adrenergic receptor by PKC-mediated phosphorylation of the α2-adrenoceptor β-subunit binding site. This may act as a negative feedback mechanism in which α1-adrenergic receptors inhibit the ability of α2-adrenergic receptors to inhibit neurotransmitter release. Finally, activation of postsynaptic β-adrenergic receptors enhances postsynaptic GABAA currents in pyramidal neurons, thereby sensitizing cortical networks to inhibitory effects (Shao et al., 2017).

a. NE is synthesized from tyrosine by hydroxylation to form dihydroxyphenylalanine (DOPA), decarboxylation to form dopamine, and hydroxylation to form NE, b.
b. and is stored in vesicles.
c. Following the appropriate stimulus (not shown), NE is released into the synaptic cleft.
d. Released NE activates adrenergic receptors located on the postsynaptic membrane (α1, β1 and β2) and
e. presynaptic membrane e (α2 and β2).
f. and causes postsynaptic reactions such as protein kinase activation and protein phosphorylation.
g. NET is responsible for NE reuptake in the synaptic cleft and terminates its operation.
h. Following re-uptake by NETs, a small proportion of NE is restored in the vesicles (following uptake by the vesicular amine transporter 2, VMAT 2);
i. the rest is metabolized in the mitochondria by the enzyme monoamine oxidase (MAO)
j. the final product, dihydroxyphenylglycol (DHPG) is released into the circulation.
k. A small proportion of synaptic NE gets into the circulation or
l. is captured by another system (Capture 2),
m. metabolized to form normetanephrine (NMN).

Since 70–90% of synaptic NE is taken up by NETs, blockade of NETs is likely to shift towards the NMN pathway and divert from the DHPG pathway. A high ratio of plasma NMN to DHPG may prove useful in measuring this blockade (Song et al., 2019).

Norepinephrine, which is a neurohormone and neurotransmitter, acts on many receptors, reducing cortical activity, either limiting the outflow of neurotransmitters, or increasing sensitivity to inhibitory signaling. Norepinephrine stimulates both α- and β-adrenergic receptors. Activation of α receptors causes vasoconstriction, increases vascular resistance and increases cardiac output. On the other hand, activated β receptors increase the contractility and excitability of the heart, and accelerate its action.

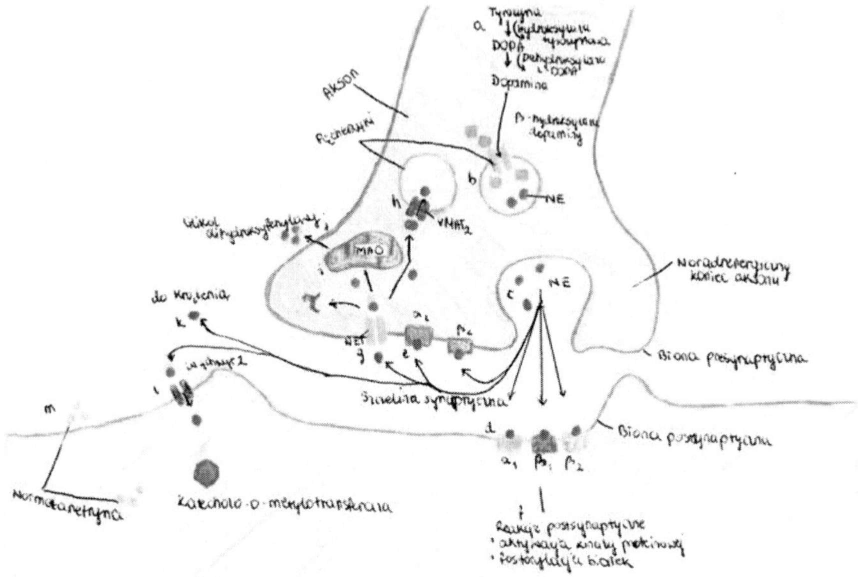

Figure 3. Diagram of noradrenergic axon terminal showing the release and reuptake of norepinephrine (NE).

References

Brown J C, Simons E, Rudders S A. Epinephrine in the Management of Anaphylaxis. *J. Allergy Clin. Immunol. Pract.* 2020 Apr;8(4):1186-1195.

Kohno R, Detloff B L, Chen L Y, Norby F L, Benditt D G. Epinephrine rise concept. *J. Cardiovasc. Electrophysiol.* 2019 Aug;30(8):1396-1397.

Shao H, Li C S. Epinephrine in Out-of-hospital Cardiac Arrest: Helpful or Harmful? *Chin. Med. J.* (Engl). 2017 Sep 5;130(17):2112-2116.

Sicherer S H, Simons F E R; Section on Allergy and Immunology. Epinephrine for First-aid Management of Anaphylaxis. *Pediatrics*. 2017 Mar;139(3): e20164006.

Song T T, Lieberman P. Who needs to carry an epinephrine autoinjector? *Cleve. Clin. J. Med.* 2019 Jan;86(1):66-72.

Chapter 21

Thyroid Hormone

Maciej Haduch, Dorota Bartusik-Aebisher*
and David Aebisher
Medical College of The University of Rzeszów, Rzeszów, Poland

Abstract

Thyroid hormones provide the body with proper metabolism thanks to which our organs function as they should, and also indirectly participate in the thermoregulation of our body. They are also very important in our immune system by acting on the appropriate receptors responsible for the transformation of monocytes into macrophages, and as a result of which it will be possible to effectively respond to microorganisms attacking our body. The thyroid gland also affects our calcium economy through the action of calcitonin, thanks to which the level of this element is not too high. It is necessary to realize the important role of the thyroid gland and its hormones in our body, as well as iodine, and be aware of serious complications caused by diseases related to disorders of the synthesis of these compounds.

Keywords: thyroid hormones, DNA, iodine, hormones, calcitonin, proteins

The thyroid hormones (thyroid Figure 1) include: calcitonin, Triiodothyronine (T3) and Thyroxine (T4). Thyroid hormones are simply responsible for the metabolism in our body and for the calcium balance in our body, but also participate in the immune response of our body.

* Corresponding Author's Email: dbartusikaebisher@ur.edu.pl.

In: The Biochemical Guide to Hormones
Editor: David Aebisher
ISBN: 979-8-88697-492-8

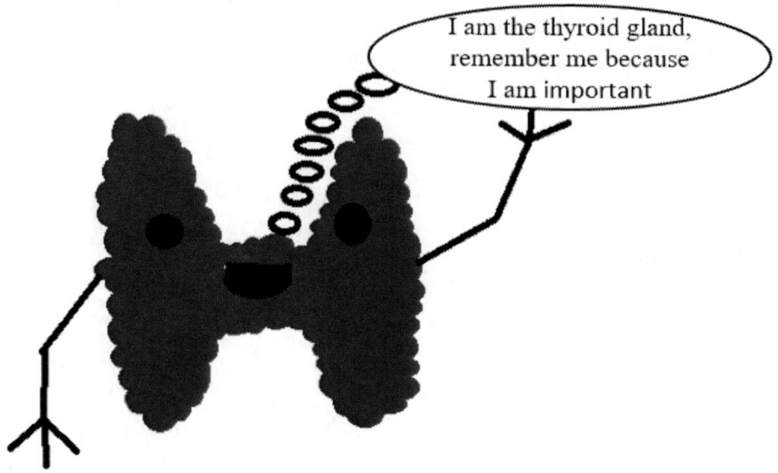
I am the thyroid gland,
remember me because
I am important

Figure 1. "The thyroid" by Maciej Haduch Description: The illustration shows the general shape of the thyroid gland.

Triiodoyronine is formed by iodination of the thyroxine molecule. It affects DNA transcription in our body and stimulates the production of ATP-dependent Na +/K + pumps, which increases the metabolism of our body. Thyroxine is made from tyrosine. It stimulates catabolic processes in our body, e.g., oxidation, as well as mental development and gonadal development. Calcitonin is made from a prohormone. This hormone is responsible for the inhibition of osteoclasts and thus the "retention" of calcium in the bones, as it will not be excreted into the blood, also affects the kidneys by reducing the excretion of calcium in our urine (Anyetei-Anum et al., 2018).

The secretion of T3 and T4 is governed by the thyroid stimulating hormone produced by the hypothalamus and is regulated in a negative-feedback fashion to the secretion of the above-mentioned. Hormones are also affected by: vasopressin, adrenaline and temperature. Calcitonin secretion is regulated by the level of calcium in the blood and glucagon (Anyetei-Anum et al., 2018).

It is a 32 amino acid polypeptide formed in the parapholic cells of the thyroid gland, necessary for the regulation of calcium and phosphorus in our body. The molecular weight is 3.42 KdA, present in our body in the form of a dimer or a monomer. This hormone is synthesized from prohormone, procalcitonin (13 kDa mass made of 116 amino acids) is an intermediate product of calcitonin synthesis and is a very important marker in infections, and more precisely its other form, which is inflammatory procalcitonin. Its expression in bacterial infections is much greater than in viral infections, because viruses inhibit its expression, thanks to this phenomenon it is possible to determine what type of pathogenic system is attacking our body. Calcitonin is responsible for reducing calcium levels in our body. This is because it inhibits the action of osteoclasts, i.e., osteogenic cells that break down our bones and introduce calcium into our body. Calcitonin can be activated by glucagon or by a high concentration of calcium or phosphorus in the plasma, which causes the increased excretion of these two elements from our body along with the urine. High levels of calcium have a negative effect on nerve cells, which is why it is important that calcitonin "keeps" its correct level in the human body (Biondi et al., 2019).

Triiodothyronine is produced in our body by de-iodination of another thyroid hormone, thyroxine, it is produced in the follicular cells of the thyroid gland. Thyroxine is also produced in follicular cells from the substrate tyrosine. These compounds provide our body with proper metabolic changes and take part in thermoregulation. Hormones act on nuclear receptors in cells, for example on cardiomyocytes. Hormones, this will affect the expression of alpha and beta isophoram proteins as well as myosin heavy chains, as well as the gene encoding ATP-a with calcium-activated sarcoplasmic reticulum, which will affect the calcium metabolism of the heart as well as his contractions and thus his metabolism. It should be noted that in target cells, thyroxine breaks down into triiodothyronine (Braun et al., 2017).

Iodine is an indispensable substrate involved in the synthesis of thyroid hormones (T3 and T4) in our body. In a slight deficiency of this element, we notice in patients the so-called Goiter, or enlargement of the thyroid gland. In severe deficiencies in children, it has been noticed that their mental state is lower than in children who do not have this deficiency. IQ tests showed that on average a person suffering from iodine deficiency, and thus triiodothyronine and thyroxine deficiency, has 13.5 points less than a healthy person (Kim et al., 2019).

There are various immune cells in our body, e.g., macrophages or lymphocytes. They are influenced by compounds from the group of cytokines that cause these cells to prevent various antigens from developing in our body. Thyroid hormones can affect our immune system by activating TRα and TRβ receptors located on the surface of min. macrophages. These hormones thus influence the process of transforming monocytes into dendritic cells by accelerating it and increasing the efficiency of phagocytosis in macrophages (Mendoza et al., 2017).

In summary, thyroid hormones are essential in our body for both the development and overall functioning of our body. They provide the body with proper metabolism, e.g., by activating the translation of genes that cause the production of SERCA pumps, thanks to which our organs function as they should, and also indirectly participate in the thermoregulation of our body (by, for example, using the above-mentioned pumps, which need ATP for their work, as a result of what the heat is generated). They are also very important in our immune system by acting on the appropriate receptors responsible for the transformation of monocytes into macrophages, and as a result of which it will be possible to effectively respond to microorganisms attacking our body, they are also a good marker of the etiology of infections, because viral infections inhibit their expression. An important fact that should also be mentioned is that these compounds play a very important role in our intellectual development, because their severe deficiency leads to significant disorders of our mind, as a result of which a child who suffered from a deficiency of thyroid hormones and thus iodine, which is necessary for their synthesis will have a relatively lower IQ by an average of 13.5 points. The thyroid gland also affects our calcium economy through the action of calcitonin, which is the excretion of $Ca2^+$ if there is too much of it in our body, thanks to which the level of this element is not too high. Bearing in mind the above-mentioned examples, it is necessary to realize the important role of the thyroid gland and its hormones in our body, as well as iodine, and be aware of serious complications caused by diseases related to disorders of the synthesis of these compounds.

References

Anyetei-Anum C. S., Roggero V. R., Allison L. A. Thyroid hormone receptor localization in target tissues. *J Endocrinol.* 2018 Apr;237(1):R19-R34.

Biondi B., Cooper D. S. Thyroid hormone therapy for hypothyroidism. *Endocrine.* 2019 Oct;66(1):18-26.

Braun D., Schweizer U. Thyroid Hormone Transport and Transporters. *Vitam Horm.* 2018;106:19-44.

Kim M. J., Park Y. J. Bisphenols and Thyroid Hormone. *Endocrinol Metab (Seoul).* 2019 Dec;34(4):340-348.

Mendoza A., Hollenberg A. N. New insights into thyroid hormone action. *Pharmacol Ther.* 2017 May;173:135-145.

Chapter 22

Ghrelin

**Klaudia Dynarowicz, Dorota Bartusik-Aebisher*
and David Aebisher**
Medical College of The University of Rzeszów, Poland

Abstract

Ghrelin is a multi-purpose intestinal peptide hormone acting as the natural agonist of the growth hormone secretagogue receptor. The main place of its production is the stomach. Ghrelin also activates the metabolism in the stomach and stimulates the process of gastric acid secretion. Ghrelin reduces the expression of pro-inflammatory cytokines, inhibits the proliferation of T lymphocytes prevents adherence of blood monocytes to vascular endothelial cells and reduces the synthesis of chemokines. Ghreli affects the process of cell proliferation and the process of apoptosis. Due to the fact that ghrelin supports the appetite, it indirectly influences body weight. Ghrelin may be an innovative therapeutic candidate for the prevention and treatment of atherosclerosis and coronary artery disease. Is a possibility of its clinical application for conditions like anorexia, cachexia, sarcopenia, gastrointestinal diseases, cardiovascular diseases, renal and pulmonary diseases, neurodegenerative disorders, inflammatory disorders and metabolic syndromes.

Keywords: ghrelin, lymphocytes, adipose tissue, atherosclerosis, growth hormone (GH), paracrine/autocrine

---

* Corresponding Author's Email: dbartusikaebisher@ur.edu.pl.

In: The Biochemical Guide to Hormones
Editor: David Aebisher
ISBN: 979-8-88697-492-8

The prefix “ghre” in ghrelin means “to grow” Ghrelin is a multi-purpose intestinal peptide hormone secreted from endocrine cells acting as the natural agonist of the growth hormone secretagogue receptor. Its molecular weight is 3315 u. The main place of its production is the stomach (Tokudome, Kangawa, 2019). It is located in the largest amounts in the submucosa.

Ghrelin was discovered in 1999. Its most visible effect is its ability to stimulate food intake. This is possible thanks to its ability to stimulate the hypothalamic nerve circuits. Ghrelin also activates the metabolism in the stomach and stimulates the process of gastric acid secretion (Poher, et al., 2018). Ghrelin secreted from the stomach stimulates the vagus nerve, transmitting a hunger signal to the brain that acts on the hypothalamic arcuate nucleus, an important region in the control of appetite. It affects many organs and glands, not only those belonging to the digestive system. Figure 1 shows the influence of ghrelin on selected organs and glands.

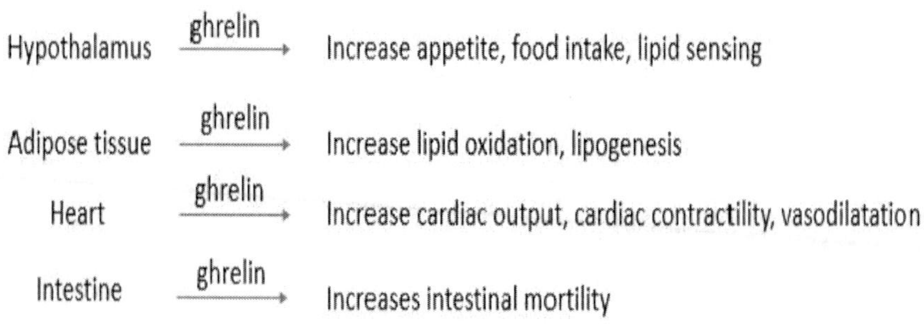

Figure 1. Influence ghrelin on selected organs or glands.

Little is known about the role of ghrelin within the pancreas, but it has been suggested that this hormone could play a paracrine/autocrine role in the regulation of β-cell survival and function. In this context, ghrelin has recently been reported to promote proliferation and cell growth and to inhibit apoptosis in a pancreatic β-cell line and human islets. Ghrelin has many beneficial and needed functions. It reduces the expression of pro-inflammatory cytokines, inhibits the proliferation of T lymphocytes prevents adherence of blood monocytes to vascular endothelial cells and reduces the synthesis of chemokines. These are just a few of its properties. Table 1 presents the most important functions of ghrelin.

Ghrelin also exhibits cardiovascular effects, mediates increases in gastric movement and gastric acid secretion, suppresses sympathetic nerve output, and contributes to the regulation of glucose metabolism. Ghrelin, produced primarily in gastrointestinal organs in response to hunger and starvation, circulates in the blood, serving as a peripheral signal telling the central nervous system to stimulate feeding. The first discoveries about ghrelin proved that this hormone is actively involved in cellular and systemic activities, including diseases and metabolic diseases. Ghrelin, among its many functions, also has the ability to control the function of neoplastic cells. It affects the process of cell proliferation and the process of apoptosis.

Table 1. Ghrelin functions

No.	Ghrelin functions
1.	Modulate hormone secretion
2.	Modulate energy balance
3.	Gastric acid release
4.	Modulate appetite
5.	Modulate gastric motility
6.	Modulate insulin secretion
7.	Body growth regulation
8.	Regulation of blood vessel tension
9.	Inhibition of aggregation of platelets and leukocytes
10	Increases local blood flow
11	Has a protective effect on the gastric and intestinal mucosa

Due to the fact that ghrelin supports the appetite, it indirectly influences body weight. During a strict diet, ghrelin levels increase. Ghrelin works by affecting cell homeostasis. According to (Spencer, et al., 2015), ghrelin influences the reactions to stress and anxiety, depression and anxiety states. Ghrelin is found in the cells of the gastric mucosa. A few years ago, a link was shown between ghrelin levels and coronary heart disease. Due to the fact that coronary artery disease is associated with atherosclerosis and the inflammatory reaction, ghrelin alleviates atherosclerosis by inhibiting endoplasmic reticulum stress. After myocardial infarction, exogenous administration of ghrelin preserves cardiac function, reduces the incidence of fatal arrhythmias, and attenuates apoptosis and ventricular remodeling, leading to improvements in heart failure. These findings suggest that ghrelin may be an innovative therapeutic candidate for the prevention and treatment of atherosclerosis and coronary artery disease. Although how ghrelin may influence the cardiovascular system is not fully understood, the cardiovascular beneficial effects are mediated possibly through a combination of various actions, such as an increase in growth hormone level, an improvement in energy balance, direct actions to the cardiovascular cells, and regulation of the autonomic nervous activity.

Additionally, ghrelin plays a significant role in regulating the electrical activity of the heart. It reduces the inducibility of ventricular tachyarrhythmias after myocardial infarction. In addition, it regulates blood pressure, which is related to the modulation of the sympathetic nervous system and the direct expansion of blood vessels. Ghrelin is a hormone that regulates numerous metabolic processes. It affects cells, tissues and organs, affecting systems and the entire body. In the future, it may become a key tool in the treatment of certain diseases. It has the potential to increase body weight and body composition through increased appetite, increased growth hormone (GH) secretion, prevention of muscle catabolism, promotion of gut motility, stimulation of gastric acid secretion, and regulation of metabolism.

These diverse actions of ghrelin raise the possibility of its clinical application for conditions like anorexia, cachexia, sarcopenia, gastrointestinal diseases, cardiovascular diseases, renal and pulmonary diseases, neurodegenerative disorders, inflammatory disorders and metabolic syndromes. Due to these and numerous other benefits of ghrelin, pharmacological targeting of the endogenous system of ghrelin is considered a promising and valuable approach for treatment of a variety of metabolic complications including cachexia associated with cancer.

References

Poher, A. L., Tschöp, M.H., Müller, T. D. Ghrelin regulation of glucose metabolism. *Peptides*, 2018, 100, 236-242.

Polińska, B., Matowicka-Karna, J., Kemona, H. The role of ghrelin in the organism. *Postepy Hig. Med. Dosw.*, 2011, 65, 1-7.

Pradhan, G., Samson, S. L., Sun, Y. Ghrelin: much more than a hunger hormone. *Curr. Opin. Clin. Nutr. Metab. Care*. 2013, 16, 619-624.

Spencer, S. J., Emmerzaal, T. L., Kozicz, T., Andrews, Z. B. Ghrelin's role in the hypothalamic-pituitary adrenal axis stress response: implications for mood disorders. *Biol. Psychiatry*. 2015, 78, 19-27.

Tokudome, T., Kangawa, K. Physiological significance of ghrelin in the cardiovascular system. *Proc. Jpn. Acad. Ser. B Phys. Bio.l Sci*. 2019, 95, 459-467.

Chapter 23

Growth Hormone Releasing Hormone (GHRH)

Karolina Radwańska, Dorota Bartusik-Aebisher[*] and David Aebisher
Medical College of The University of Rzeszów, Rzeszów, Poland

Abstract

GHRH (Growth hormone releasing hormone) is a hormone whose main task is to release growth hormone (GH) and stimulate its synthesis in the anterior pituitary gland. GHRH deficiency or impaired synthesis is the direct cause of GH deficiency. Not only does it play an endocrine role in the body, it also controls the process of apoptosis, proliferation, survival and cell differentiation. The cause of GHRH-related abnormalities may be both its deficiency in the blood, as well as the mutation of the GHRH gene causing the autosomal recessive IGHD disease, which results in disturbances in the growth process visible already in the first year of the child's life. Studies also show a decrease in the activity of the fibrinolytic system, which can cause blood clots. Thanks to the discovery of the direct influence of GHRH on GH levels, it was possible to implement anti-cancer therapy consisting in blocking the GHRH receptor with its antagonists. This procedure is one of the methods of alternative therapy for pancreatic, stomach or colon cancer.

Keywords: growth hormone releasing hormone (GHRH), receptors, apoptosis, proliferation, growth hormone (GH)

---

[*] Corresponding Author's Email: dbartusikaebisher@ur.edu.pl.

In: The Biochemical Guide to Hormones
Editor: David Aebisher
ISBN: 979-8-88697-492-8

GHRH (Growth hormone releasing hormone) is a hormone produced by the hypothalamus, released into the portal circulation of the pituitary gland, whose main task is to release GH and stimulate its synthesis in the anterior pituitary gland. GHRH deficiency or impaired synthesis is the direct cause of GH deficiency. However, GHRH cannot be treated as an indicator of the study of the somatotrophic function of the pituitary gland due to the extreme variability of GHRH levels in healthy people. The presence of GHRH, as well as its receptors, has been demonstrated both in the pituitary gland and in peripheral tissues. Not only does it play an endocrine role in the body, it also controls the process of apoptosis, proliferation, survival and cell differentiation. GHRH also affects skeletal muscle cells, wound healing, reducing inflammation, the functioning of pancreatic islets, β cells, and the reproductive system. The mechanism of action of GHRH on peripheral extra-pituitary tissues is not fully understood, and the identification of extra-pituitary receptors of this hormone is difficult. GHRH is presumed to be not only endocrine but also paracrine and autocrine in nature (Barabuti et al. 2020).

The cause of GHRH-related abnormalities may be both its deficiency in the blood (the direct cause of the decrease in GH levels causing, among others, a decrease in muscle mass), as well as the mutation of the GHRH gene causing the autosomal recessive IGHD disease, which results in disturbances in the growth process visible already in the first year of the child's life. GHRH is synthesized in the hypothalamic neurons, located in the arcuate and ventrolateral nuclei. Growth hormone releasing hormone acts on the pituitary gland to stimulate the production and release of growth hormone as well as the proliferation of the pituitary cells themselves. The actions of GHRH are made possible by the GHRH receptors, belonging to B-III, which belong to the superfamily of G protein-coupled receptors. GHRH receptor gene expression is regulated by glucocorticoids (Lim et al. 2018).

The role of GHRH in releasing growth hormone is well known, however, the hormone has a much broader spectrum of activity in peripheral tissue cells. The content of GHRH was detected in the secretions of the duodenum, stomach, liver, lung, jejunum, pancreas, as well as in the cells of the kidney, prostate, breast, thymus and cells of the immune system. GHRH stimulates insulin secretion by pancreatic β-cells as well as pancreatic digestive enzymes. Its high concentration has been observed not only in normal pancreatic cells, but also in their cancer cells. The hormone also affects the reproductive system. It has been proven that GHRH stimulates the maturation of reproductive cells and enables the production of hormones in the testes and ovaries (the presence of GHRH receptors has also been observed in the gonads) (Lim e et al. 2018).

GHRH affects muscle function and the respiratory capacity of the body. Scientists have found that deficiency of this hormone causes an impairment of oxygen uptake by skeletal muscle cells. The dysfunction of the muscular system is also associated with abnormal work of the circulatory system and reduced ability to sweat, which reduces exercise capacity. The reason for the abnormal functioning of blood vessels, related to GHRH deficiency, is often coronary artery disease, caused by a reduced content of HDL in patients, as well as an increase in the deposition of cholesterol on the walls of the vessels. Studies also show a decrease in the activity of the fibrinolytic system, which can cause blood clots. A decrease in the concentration of GHRH or its incorrect synthesis leads to a deficiency of growth hormone (GH). The abnormality may be acquired as a result of damage to the hypothalamus or congenital, caused by organic changes. This condition inhibits the growth and development of children's skeletons. Recent studies have substantiated the unfounded view that the decline in GHRH levels in adults would not be consistent. It has been proven that the deficiency of the above-mentioned hormone results in worse health, shorter survival time, a decrease in the concentration of IgF-I in the plasma, as well as an increased incidence of cardiovascular diseases. In addition, the direct cause of the decline in GH levels is a decline in the production of GHRH by the hypothalamus due to aging (Sanchez Jimenez et al. 2021).

GHRH deficiency may also have a genetic basis (IGHD disease). The reason for the decrease in the hormone concentration is a homozygous mutation of the receptor. Sick people have a very low concentration of IgF-I in the plasma and are characterized by short stature. Additional symptoms associated with the receptor mutation are obesity, high voice and wrinkled skin. An interesting phenomenon is the appearance of "youthful hair" that practically does not turn gray. In newborns with the disease, IGHD symptoms cannot be observed, which confirms the thesis that GHRH is not necessary for proper intrauterine growth (Yuen et al. 2019).

Immunoreactive GHRH is present not only in neoplastic cells of the pancreas, but also in carcinoid tumors, small cell lung cancer, adrenal adenomas, tumors of the stomach, brain, prostate, and ovary. An interesting fact is the lack of increased GHRH parameters in the peripheral blood in patients with hypothalamic tumors, although the secretion of this hormone is much higher. This is due to the direct delivery of GHRH produced in the hypothalamus to the portal pituitary system, bypassing the systemic circulation. One of the symptoms of GHRH-secreting peripheral tumors is an enlargement of the pituitary gland. GHRH has also been detected in malignant neoplasms such as ovarian and breast cancer (Zhang et al. 2020).

Growth hormone releasing hormone has many functions in the body. It works not only on GH, but is also present in the cells of the pancreas, reproductive cells and the breast. It enables the proper proliferation of cells, the synthesis of gonadotropins, and also influences muscle function and skeletal development. Both its deficiency and mutations in the coding gene have serious consequences and cause disease. Research on the understanding of the mechanism of action of GHRH allowed for a breakthrough discovery that contributed to the fight against malignant tumors. The formation and release of GH requires an earlier interaction of GHRH with receptors located in the membrane of somatotropic cells in the anterior pituitary gland. Investigation of the growth hormone releasing hormone pathway was made possible by the identification of these receptors (family B-III coupled with G protein). The GHRH receptor signals mainly via cAMP-dependent pathways (Zhang et al. 2020). Thanks to the discovery of the direct influence of GHRH on GH levels, it was possible to implement anti-cancer therapy consisting in blocking the GHRH receptor with its antagonists. This procedure is one of the methods of alternative therapy for pancreatic, stomach or colon cancer. Thanks to this, the agonists have anti-proliferative, anti-metastatic and anti-angiogenic properties.

References

Barabutis N. A glimpse at growth hormone-releasing hormone cosmos. *Clin. Exp. Pharmacol. Physiol.* 2020 Sep;47(9):1632-1634.

Lim CT, Korbonits M. Update on the Clinicopathology of Pituitary Adenomas. *Endocr. Pract.* 2018 May;24(5):473-488.

Sanchez Jimenez JG, De Jesus O. Hypothalamic Dysfunction. 2021 Aug 30. In: StatPearls [Internet]. *Treasure Island* (FL): StatPearls Publishing; 2021 Jan- .PMID: 32809578.

Yuen KCJ, Biller BMK, Radovick S, Carmichael JD, Jasim S, Pantalone KM, Hoffman AR. American association of clinical endocrinologists and American college of endocrinology guidelines for management of growth hormone deficiency in adults and patients transitioning from pediatric to adult care. *Endocr. Pract.* 2019 Nov;25(11):1191-1232.

Zhang C, Cui T, Cai R, Wangpaichitr M, Mirsaeidi M, Schally AV, Jackson RM. Growth Hormone-Releasing Hormone in Lung Physiology and Pulmonary Disease. *Cells.* 2020 Oct 21;9(10):2331.

Chapter 24

Thyrotropin Releasing Hormone (TRH)

Patrycja Patronik, Dorota Bartusik-Aebisher*
and David Aebisher
Medical College of The University of Rzeszów, Poland

Abstract

Thyreoliberin is an important peptide hormone that is responsible for many numerous processes in the body. TRH and its analogues have a significantly shorter half-life, longer duration of effects, and little development of tolerance after prolonged dosing. By acting as an anticonvulsant and suppressing memory impairment, it sheds new light on the treatment of diseases such as Parkinson's disease and Alzheimer's disease, which is of great clinical importance. Disorders on the hypothalamic-pituitary-thyroid axis controlled by it can be the source of many diseases such as hyperthyroidism and hypothyroidism. Due to the variety and scale of activity, thyreoliberin and its analogues are still an interesting subject of research.

Keywords: thyrotropin releasing hormone (TRH), Parkinson's disease, Alzheimer's disease, hypophysiotropic hormone

Thyreoliberin (TRH) is a hypothalamic hormone belonging to liberin, synthesized in the hypothalamus, which is the link between the central nervous system, and the pituitary gland, the work of which is controlled by Figure 1 The exact place of its production is the paraventricular nucleus of the

* Corresponding Author's Email: dbartusikaebisher@ur.edu.pl.

In: The Biochemical Guide to Hormones
Editor: David Aebisher
ISBN: 979-8-88697-492-8

hypothalamus (PVN), apart from it, it can be formed in various locations of the central nervous system and in secretory organs, e.g., spinal cord, hippocampus, cortex of the brain, β- cells pancreas and testes This neuropeptide reaches the pituitary gland through the portal system of vessels, more specifically to its anterior lobe and stimulates the secretion of thyrotropin (TSH) by it. TSH stimulates the thyroid gland to secrete the hormones triiodothyronine (T3) and thyroxine (T4) responsible for controlling the speed of the course of many metabolic changes in all cells of the body (Al-Chalabi et al., 2021).

TRH secretion is controlled by neurotransmitters, norepinephrine stimulates this process, and dopamine is inhibitory. From the above information, we can conclude that TRH controls the hypothalamic-pituitary-thyroid neuroendocrine axis on the basis of a negative feedback loop. When the concentration of T3 and T4 hormones increases in the body, the secretion of TSH and TRH is inhibited. TRH has a much wider spectrum of activity, one of them is its involvement in the production and release of hormones such as prolactin, growth hormone, and insulin or vasopressin, and also the neurotransmitters belonging to the central nervous system – noradrenaline and adrenaline, and also controls the homeostasis of the CNS. Due to the wide range of functions and their essence, any disorders related to TRH secretion significantly affect other cells of the body (Bowden et al., 2021).

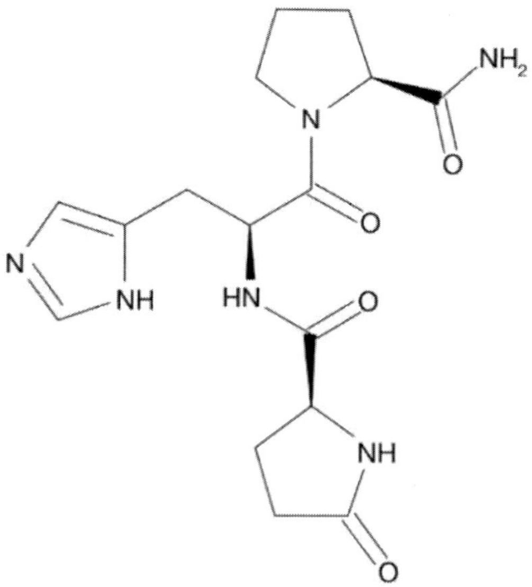

Figure 1. Structural formula of Thyreoliberin. [Own study].

The history of the discovery of the thyrotropin releasing hormone dates back to the 1930s. It was then discovered that there was a connection between the pituitary gland and the hypothalamus through the transport of substances. The peptide structure of the pituitary gland hormones was determined in 1969, when its proper structure was discovered by the French-American neurobiologist Roger Guillemin and Andrew V. Schally, an American endocrinologist of Polish origin. In 1977 their work was awarded the Nobel Prize in Medicine "for their discoveries in the production of peptide hormones in the brain." This discovery made it possible to learn about many new peptides produced by the pituitary gland, and also allowed for the development of further research opening new, unknown perspectives in medicine. Thyreoliberin, a hypophysiotropic hormone with a molecular weight of 359.9 Da, has the structure of (pyro) Glu-His-Pro-NH2 and is produced as a result of post-translational processing of a large precursor protein, the biosynthesis of which depends on the regulation of thyroid hormone feedback, the influence of the central nervous system, and also stimulants and inhibitors The secretagogues include:

- Long-term emotions,
- Sleep,
- Cold,
- The factors that inhibit secretion include, among others:
- Stress,
- Heat,
- Increase in the concentration of T_3 and T_4 hormones,
- Stimulating the secretion of hormones (Mathew et al., 2021).

The activity of thyreoliberin depends on the time of day, it occurs during the night to the most intense secretory process. Cold acts on thermoreceptors, stimulating the secretion of TRH by the hypothalamus, so that in winter its activity as well as hormones secreted on the hypothalamic-pituitary-thyroid axis will be much greater than in summer. Stress is a factor that affects both the limbic system and the pituitary gland by inhibiting the secretion of hormones. Increase in hormone levels T3 and T4 works on the principle of negative feedback, in the case of too active secretion of these hormones by the thyroid gland, the activity of the anterior pituitary gland and the paraventricular nucleus of the hypothalamus is reduced Figure 2. On the other hand, heat acts antagonistically to cold, inhibiting the secretory process.

Adrenocorticotropic hormones and glucocorticoids also have an inhibitory effect. An important site of TRH action is the brainstem and the level of the midbrain, this is where the regulation of food and water intake takes place, which is inhibited by the action of TRH, which is why it was considered to be used in the treatment of obesity (Shahid et al., 2021).

TRH activating successive hormones in a cascade is responsible for metabolic processes occurring throughout the body, and also maintains homeostasis in thermoregulatory centers. One of the most important and widely documented effects of this peptide hormone of the hypothalamus is its antidepressant effect, and it also shows beneficial effects in the treatment of bipolar disorder. TRH is involved in the alleviation of seizures, and these data provide grounds for its potential use as an adjuvant in epileptic states. However, it is not the only disease in which the use of TRH is considered as a drug, because it is also in neurodegenerative diseases such as Alzheimer's disease or Parkinsonh's disease. TRH was also used for diagnostic purposes, to diagnose classic hyperthyroidism, but it was replaced by the ultrasensitive TSH test method. The TRH stimulation test is still an important aspect in the diagnosis of congenital central hypothyroidism, which enables a rapid therapeutic response. A special analogue is taltireline, which can be used in the treatment of depressive diseases because it stimulates the release of dopamine and controls the regulation of the sympathetic nervous system (Singh et al., 2019).

Thyreoliberin is an important peptide hormone that is responsible for many numerous processes in the body, as well as offers new therapeutic possibilities in the treatment and diagnosis of diseases. TRH and its analogues have a significantly shorter half-life, longer duration of effects, and little development of tolerance after prolonged dosing. In Japan, one of the thyreoliberin analogues, Talitrelin, has already been approved as a drug for spinocerebellar degeneration in the form of a drug called Ceredist. By acting as an anticonvulsant and suppressing memory impairment, it sheds new light on the treatment of diseases such as Parkinson's disease and Alzheimer's disease, which is of great clinical importance. Disorders on the hypothalamic-pituitary-thyroid axis controlled by it can be the source of many diseases such as hyperthyroidism and hypothyroidism. TRH inhibits the release of vasopressin and oxytocin, the above examples confirm its role as a neurotransmitter or neuromodulator in the central nervous system involved in many regulatory processes. The activity of the synthesis and secretion of this hormone is influenced both by external conditions beyond our control, such as the temperature dictated by the seasons of the year, and factors such as stress or regular sleep of a sufficiently long duration, as well as the state of our health. Therefore, it is important to take care of sleep hygiene and minimize stress factors on our body. Due to the variety and scale of activity, thyreoliberin and its analogues are still an interesting subject of research.

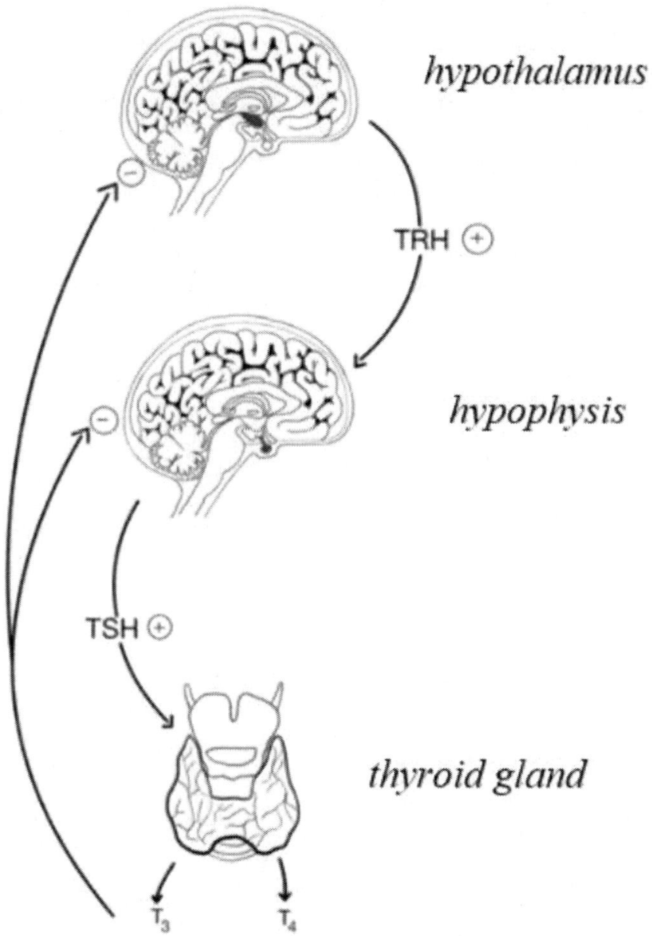

Figure 2. Regulation of the neuroendocrine axis according to the principle of negative feedback. [Own study].

References

Al-Chalabi M, Bass A N, Alsalman I. *Physiology, Prolactin*. 2021 Jul 29. In: StatPearls [Internet]. Treasure Island (FL): StatPearls Publishing; 2021 Jan–.PMID: 29939606.

Bowden S A, Goldis M. *Congenital Hypothyroidism*. 2021 Aug 2. In: StatPearls [Internet]. Treasure Island (FL): StatPearls Publishing; 2021 Jan–. PMID: 32644339.

Clarias batrachus and its role in regulation of hypophysiotropic dopamine neurons. *J. Comp. Neurol*. 2019 Apr 15;527(6):1070-1101.

Mathew P, Rawla P. *Hyperthyroidism*. 2021 Jul 9. In: StatPearls [Internet]. Treasure Island (FL): StatPearls Publishing; 2021 Jan–. PMID: 30725738.

Shahid M A, Ashraf M A, Sharma S. *Physiology, Thyroid Hormone*. 2021 May 12. In: StatPearls [Internet]. Treasure Island (FL): StatPearls Publishing; 2021 Jan–. PMID: 29763182.

Singh O, Pradhan D R, Nagalakashmi B, Kumar S, Mitra S, Sagarkar S, Sakharkar A J, Lechan RM, Singru PS. *Thyrotropin-releasing hormone (TRH) in the brain and pituitary of the teleost.*

Chapter 25

Gonadotropin Releasing Hormone (GnRH)

**Maja Mularczyk, Dorota Bartusik-Aebisher*
and David Aebisher**
Medical College of The University of Rzeszów, Poland

Abstract

Gonadoliberin, a hormone synthesized by the hypothalamus and controls the synthesis of lutropin and follicle stimulating hormone. GnRH is a factor that should be checked in the case of ovulation disorders in a woman. In the case of menstruation disorders or problems with becoming pregnant, the level of luteinizing hormone and follicle stimulating hormone should be checked. In the case of fertility treatment, your doctor may prescribe gonadotrophin treatment. This treatment is selected for patients with impaired functioning of the hypothalamic-pituitary system. Lack of sexual maturity in children and non-production of secondary sexual characteristics may be a signal that the secretion of hormones: GnRH, LH and FSH is disturbed. That is why it is very important to control your gonadoliberin levels at every stage of your life.

Keywords: gonadotropin releasing hormone (GnRH), follicle stimulating hormone (FSH), hormones, lutropin (LH), testosteron, estrogen

Gonadoliberin is an extremely important hormone made of just 10 amino acids. It is produced and secreted by specialized nerve cells in the hypothalamus. It is then released into small blood vessels that carry the

* Corresponding Author's Email: dbartusikaebisher@ur.edu.pl.

In: The Biochemical Guide to Hormones
Editor: David Aebisher
ISBN: 979-8-88697-492-8

hormone to the pituitary gland. GnRH acts on the anterior pituitary gland, stimulating the synthesis and release of gonadotrophins: lutropin (LH) and follicle stimulating hormone (FSH). These hormones are extremely important to the reproductive health of both women and men. The release of these hormones is feedback-controlled. Gonadoliberin is degraded by proteolysis within minutes (Barabás et al., 2020).

During childhood, GnRH levels are low. As puberty approaches, the gonadotropin releasing hormone increases, which causes the onset of sexual maturation. When the testes and ovaries are fully developed, the production of GnRH, LH and FSH is controlled by the levels of testosterone and the female sex hormones (estrogen and progesterone). If the level of these hormones increases, the production of GnRH decreases and vice versa (Figure 2). GnRH secretion is different in men and women. In men, gonadoliberin is excreted by pulses at a constant frequency, and in women, the frequency of the pulses changes during the menstrual cycle, and just before ovulation we observe a large increase in GnRH. A GnRH deficiency in childhood means that a person is not going through adolescence. An example is the rare Kallman syndrome, which causes loss of development of the nerve cells that produce gonadoliberin, resulting in a loss of puberty (Barabás et al., 2020).

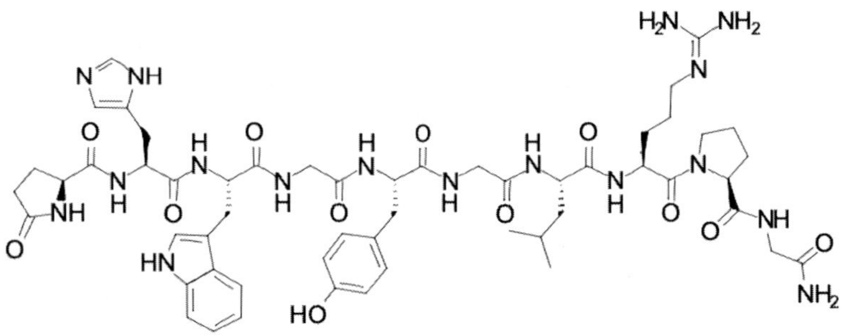

Figure 1. Structural formula of Gonadoliberin. [Own study].

Gonadoliberin is a very necessary hormone in the maturation process, the menstrual cycle and the process of spermatogenesis. Due to the occurrence of these processes, a woman and a man are fertile. Well, the menstrual cycle that we observe in a woman's body is the result of a complex exchange of information between the hypothalamus, pituitary gland, ovaries and the uterus. Although women often complain about these few days a month they realize that this is an inevitable process leading to motherhood. The menstrual cycle is under the control of hormones, the most important of which are:

- GnRH – gonadoliberin,
- FSH – follicle stimulating hormone,
- LH – lutropin,
- Estrogen.

Gonadoliberin stimulates the pituitary gland to synthesize LH and FSH. Increasing levels of follicle stimulating hormone in the blood allow immature follicles to develop in both ovaries. It is thanks to her that the Graaf follicle develops in the ovaries. When you get inadequate FSH levels, your follicles may not develop properly. Even a slight change in LH and FSH levels can cause cycle abnormalities leading to anovulation. As is well known, ovulation means the release of an oocyte ready for fertilization. In its absence, there is no possibility of fertilization. The proper production of female sex hormones requires stimulation with both gonadotrophins. When sufficient estrogen levels are reached in the blood, FSH production is inhibited. Estrogen stimulates the secretion of LH, allowing the Graaf's follicle to transform into a corpus luteum, which produces progesterone to prepare the uterus to accept an embryo. Gonadoliberin and its ability to stimulate the pituitary gland can often be the key to the formation of life. These three hormones (GnRH, FSH, LH) are the key to proper ovulation (Kittai et al., 2018).

Nowadays, young and middle-aged men reach for testosterone preparations. They are concerned about symptoms such as decreased libido or erectile dysfunction. Unfortunately, these preparations can negatively affect the hypothalamic-pituitary-gonadal axis, which can cause spermatogenesis disorders (the process of formation and maturation of male gametes – sperm). Testosterone synthesis is regulated by the hypothalamic-pituitary system. GnRH stimulates the pituitary to secrete LH. Lutropin stimulates the Leydig cells in the testes to produce testosterone. When testosterone levels rise, the secretion of gonadoliberin and lutropin is inhibited by feedback. That is why you should not "take shortcuts," that is, use testosterone preparations right away, but find out why we do not have enough of it. Maybe there's a problem with the hypothalamus not releasing the right amount of gonadoliberin? Or maybe the problem is the pituitary gland, which releases too little lutropin? If you want to use the preparation with testosterone, you should consult your doctor first. Unjustified use of testosterone may cause hypogonadism and impaired fertility in men (Tzoupis et al., 2020).

GnRH deficiency causes a reduction in the level of sex hormones, which leads to a lack of sexual maturity and non-production of secondary sexual characteristics. Childhood gonadoliberin deficiency may be due to Kallman syndrome. The disease may be inherited or spontaneous. This syndrome is much more common in men who have small testicles or cryptorchidism. In the case of the disease in women, we do not observe breast development. This disease is often accompanied by an impaired sense of smell. In adults, hypogonadotrophic hypogonadism is diagnosed with low LH and FSH levels, with low testosterone levels in men, and low levels of estradiol in women (Stamatiades et al., 2018).

Gonadoliberin analogues are a group of drugs that inhibit the release of gonadoliberin, which results in the inhibition of the release of lutropin and follicle stimulating hormone. These drugs are used in gynecology and oncology they cause pharmacological castration. They are used in the treatment of breast cancer and prostate cancer (Whitlock et al., 2019).

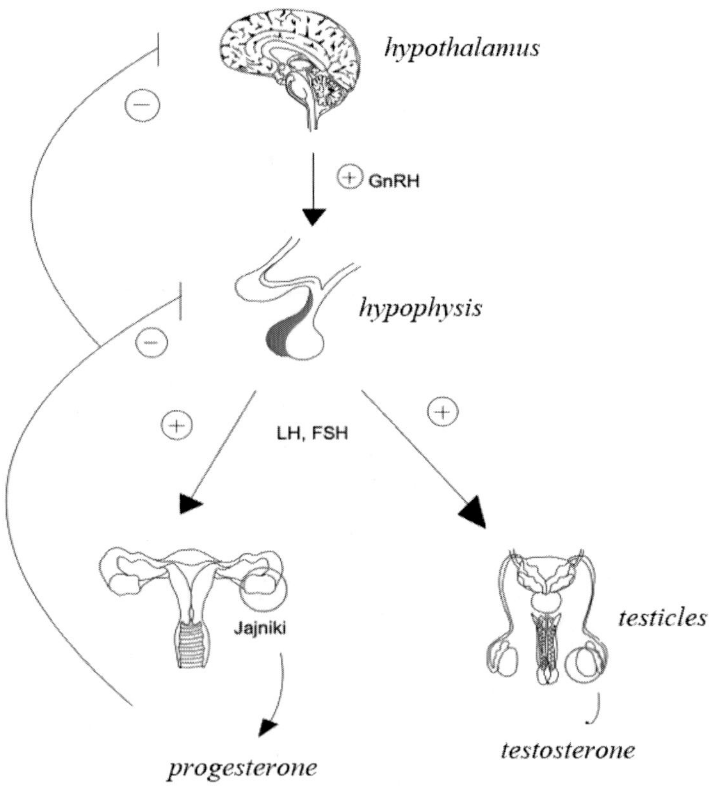

Figure 2. Regulation of the hypothalamic-pituitary-gonadal axis by negative feedback. [Own study].

Gonadoliberin, a hormone synthesized by the hypothalamus controls the synthesis of lutropin and follicle stimulating hormone by the anterior pituitary gland. This control is very important for the body of a woman and a man.

GnRH is a factor that should be checked in the case of ovulation disorders in a woman. Limiting its release disturbs the control of FSH and LH synthesis. Both of these hormones are extremely important when planning a pregnancy. In the ovary, they stimulate the growth and maturation of the egg cells, and the formation and development of the corpus luteum, which is essential for the maintenance of pregnancy. In the case of menstruation disorders or problems with becoming pregnant, the level of luteinizing hormone and follicle stimulating hormone should be checked. In the case of fertility treatment, your doctor may prescribe gonadotrophin treatment. This treatment is selected for patients with impaired functioning of the hypothalamic-pituitary system. In men, insufficient control of LH synthesis by gonadoliberin may impair the testosterone synthesis process and, consequently, disturb the spermatogenesis process. This may result in abnormal sperm parameters. In the case of low-quality sperm, there may be sperm with abnormal mobility and shape, which is the cause of male infertility.

Lack of sexual maturity in children and non-production of secondary sexual characteristics may be a signal that the secretion of hormones: GnRH, LH and FSH is disturbed. That is why it is very important to control your gonadoliberin levels at every stage of your life. Its proper control of release has given many people the happiness that comes from proper maturation as well as the possibility of having children.

References

Barabás K, Szabó-Meleg E, Ábrahám I M. Effect of Inflammation on Female Gonadotropin-Releasing Hormone (GnRH) Neurons: Mechanisms and Consequences. *Int. J. Mol. Sci.* 2020 Jan 14;21(2):529.

Kittai A S, Blank J, Graff J N. Gonadotropin-Releasing Hormone Antagonists in Prostate Cancer. *Oncology* (Williston Park). 2018 Dec 17;32(12):599-602, 604-6. PMID: 30632129.

Stamatiades G A, Kaiser U B. Gonadotropin regulation by pulsatile GnRH: Signaling and gene expression. *Mol. Cell Endocrinol.* 2018 Mar 5;463:131-141.

Tzoupis H, Nteli A, Androutsou M E, Tselios T. Gonadotropin-Releasing Hormone and GnRH Receptor: Structure, Function and Drug Development. *Curr. Med. Chem.* 2020;27(36):6136-6158.

Whitlock K E, Postlethwait J, Ewer J. Neuroendocrinology of reproduction: Is gonadotropin-releasing hormone (GnRH) dispensable? *Front Neuroendocrinol.* 2019 Apr;53:100738.

Chapter 26

Corticotropin Releasing Hormone (CRH)

**Gabriela Pinkowska, Dorota Bartusik-Aebisher*
and David Aebisher**
Medical College of The University of Rzeszów, Rzeszów, Poland

Abstract

Corticoliberin is a peptide that plays a fundamental role in coordinating the neuroendocrine-immune response to stress. It affects the regulation of the feeling of hunger (appetite) in the body and affects the duration of pregnancy, as well as the delivery itself. Its increased amount may stimulate the mechanisms leading to the occurrence of depression and anxiety disorders. In recent years, the knowledge about the complex regulatory mechanisms of corticoliberin activity, including new directions of action of this neuropeptide in the human body, has increased significantly. Understanding its distribution in the central nervous system enables its function as a neurotransmitter and neuromodulator to be determined.

Keywords: corticotropin releasing hormone (CRH), Alzheimer's disease, corticoliberin, hypothalamic-pituitary-adrenal (HPA)

Corticoliberin (corticotropin releasing hormone, CRH) is a multi-peptide-releasing neurotransmitter, belonging to the family of corticotropin releasing factors. In humans, it is encoded by the CRH gene. It was first isolated and discovered from over 500,000 sheep hypothalamus in 1981. They then discovered a number of CRH-related peptides and receptors in vertebrates and

* Corresponding Author's Email: dbartusikaebisher@ur.edu.pl.

In: The Biochemical Guide to Hormones
Editor: David Aebisher
ISBN: 979-8-88697-492-8

invertebrates. Its main function is to stimulate the pituitary ACTH (corticotropin) synthesis in the HPA axis (hypothalamic-pituitary-adrenal) (Battaglia et al., 2020). Corticotropin Releasing Hormone (CRH) is a 41 amino acid peptide derived from 196 amino acid preprohormone. Corticoliberin is secreted in response to stress by the supraventricular nucleus (PVN) of the hypothalamus and then enters the pituitary gland via portal pituitary circulation. Increased CRH production has been reported to be associated with Alzheimer's disease and major depression, and autosomal hypothalamic hypothalamic corticotropin deficiency has numerous metabolic and potentially fatal consequences, including hypoglycemia. In addition to being produced in the hypothalamus, CRH is also synthesized in peripheral tissues such as T lymphocytes and is highly expressed in the placenta. In the placenta, CRH is an indicator of the length of pregnancy, and the duration of labor and delivery. Rapid increase in CRH concentration is present in the circulation early in labor, suggesting that in addition to its metabolic function, CRH may act as a labor enhancer. CRH is also involved in the regulation of appetite, and its administration to the central nervous system inhibits it (Battaglia et al., 2020).

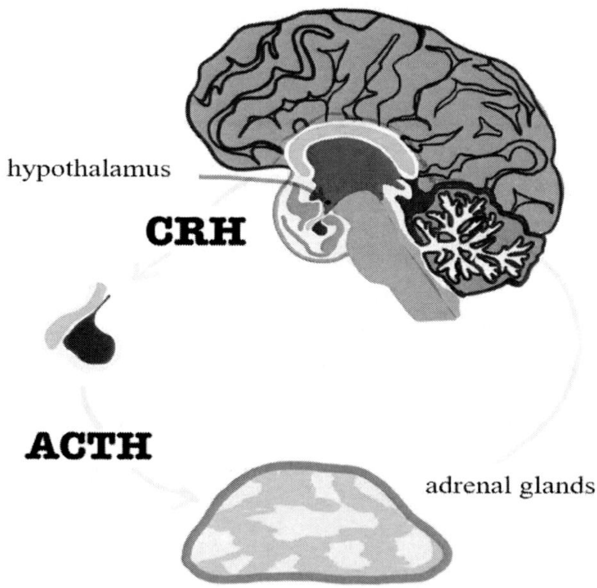

Figure 1. Shows the hypothalamic-pituitary-adrenal axis, which is mediated by corticotropin releasing hormone (CRH) and which acts on a negative feedback basis to keep the hormones involved in it constant.

Corticoliberin is produced by small cell neuroendocrine cells in the ventral tegmental area of the hypothalamus and is released into the primary capillary plexus of the portal hypothalamic-pituitary system. The portal system carries CRH to the anterior pituitary gland, where it stimulates corticotropic factors to secrete adrenocorticotropic hormone (ACTH) and other biologically active substances, i.e., β-endorphins. ACTH stimulates the synthesis of cortisol, glucocorticoids, mineralocorticosteroids and dehydroepiandrosterone (Cardoso et al., 2020). In the short term, CRH can suppress the feeling of hunger and an increased desire to provide food to the body, increase the feeling of anxiety and perform other functions such as increased concentration. While the target effects of corticoliberin are immunosuppressive through the effects of cortisol, CRH alone may actually exacerbate inflammation in the process being studied in multiple sclerosis research. The CRH1 receptor opponent, pexacerfont, is currently under investigation for the treatment of generalized anxiety disorders. Another CRH1 opponent, antalarmine, has been tested in animals for the treatment of anxiety and depression and other mental conditions, but no human studies have been conducted with this compound. In addition, nontyopic increased levels of CRH were detected in the cerebrospinal fluid of people who committed suicide. Recent studies have linked CRH1 receptor activation to alcohol euphoria. The CRH1 receptor antagonist developed by Pfizer, CP-154,526, is being investigated as a potential treatment for alcoholism. CRH is also synthesized by the placenta and appears to determine the duration of pregnancy (Cardoso et al., 2020). The level of this hormone increases in late pregnancy, just before delivery, and the current theory suggests three roles of CRH during labor: it increases dehydroepiandrosterone directly by acting on the adrenal glands, fetal kidneys and indirectly via the maternal pituitary gland; DHEA plays a role in preparing and stimulating cervical contractions, increasing the availability of prostaglandins in uterine cell tissues; prostaglandins induce contractions of the cervix, before delivery, they can act as contraction inhibitors by increasing the level of cAMP in the uterine muscle. Corticoliberin is suppressed by progesterone and remains elevated throughout pregnancy. Its release is stimulated by glucocorticoids and catecholamines, which increase before birth, reducing the blockage of progesterone (Sanchez Jimenez et al., 2021). Studies in mammals have shown that CRH has no significant stimulatory effect on the thyroid hormone. However, in all non-mammalian vertebrates, CRH has been found to have a potent thyrotropic function in addition to a corticotropic function, working with thyreoliberin to control the thyroid axis (TRH has been shown to be less effective than CRH in some species). Corticotropin-releasing hormone has been shown to interact with corticotropin-releasing hormone 1 (CRFR1) receptors and corticotropin-releasing hormone 2 (CRFR2) to produce their effects. Injection of CRF into the ventral striatum of the hypothalamus of rodents (PVN) can increase the expression of CRFR1, with the increased expression leading to behavior similar to mental disorders such as depression (Sanchez Jimenez et al., 2021). Sex differences were also observed in the case of CRF and the receptors with which it interacts. CRFR1 has been found to be present at higher levels in the female nucleus, olfactory bulb, and anterior ventral nucleus (AVPV) than in male hamsters, while male hamsters show elevated levels of CRFR2 in the terminal striatum compared to male hamsters with babies. The CRH stimulation test performed is the standard hypothalamic-pituitary-adrenal (HPA) axis challenge test used to check the activity of the hypothalamic CRH nervous system (Yi et al., 2021). Administering CRH to humans causes ACTH to be released rapidly into the bloodstream, followed by the release of cortisol and other adrenal steroids, including aldosterone. Since CRH in humans and sheep appears to have the same diagnostic value, most studies have used sheep CRH, which is more potent and longer-acting than human CRH. The test is done by injecting 100 micrograms or 1 microgram/kg of CRH into a vein. The maximum ACTH response is activated after 30 minutes and the cortisol peak (above 20 micrograms/dL) is activated after 60 minutes. Despite the large variability in the body's response to ACTH, a corticoliberin stimulation test may be useful in demonstrating adrenocorticotropic hormone deficiency or Cushing's disease (Zhang et al., 2020).

More than 20 years after the biochemical characterization of corticoliberin and the subsequent development of a specific radioactivity test, the hormone remains a promising diagnostic tool under behavioral and reproductive conditions. It has not yet entered clinical practice as a routine diagnostic marker, but rather as a pharmacological stimulus to evaluate ACTH release from the pituitary gland. Corticoliberin is a peptide that plays a fundamental role in coordinating the neuroendocrine-immune response to stress. Released from the hypothalamus into the portal circulation of the pituitary gland, it initiates the activation of the hypothalamic-pituitary axis of the adrenal glands. It affects the regulation of the feeling of hunger (appetite) in the body and affects the duration of pregnancy, as well as the delivery itself. Its increased amount may stimulate the mechanisms leading to the occurrence of depression and anxiety disorders. In recent years, the knowledge about the complex regulatory mechanisms of corticoliberin activity, including new directions of action of this neuropeptide in the human body, has increased significantly. CRH was originally known as a peptide found in the hypothalamic-pituitary system. Understanding its distribution in the central nervous system enables its function as a neurotransmitter and neuromodulator to be determined. The identification of the two corticoliberin receptors and distinct ligands contributed to a new view of the neuroendocrine stress response and related behaviors. These findings, as well as the generation of genetic models characterized by inappropriate or missing expression of individual components of the CRH system, revealed important new aspects of the corticoliberin pathway that was previously unknown or not fully understood.

References

Battaglia C. R., Cursano S., Calzia E., Catanese A., Boeckers T. M. Corticotropin-releasing hormone (CRH) alters mitochondrial morphology and function by activating the NF-kB-DRP1 axis in hippocampal neurons. *Cell Death Dis.* 2020 Nov 23;11(11):1004.

Cardoso J. C. R., Bergqvist C. A., Larhammar D. Corticotropin-Releasing Hormone (CRH) Gene Family Duplications in Lampreys Correlate With Two Early Vertebrate Genome Doublings. *Front Neurosci.* 2020 Jul 30;14:672.

Sanchez Jimenez J. G., De Jesus O. Hypothalamic Dysfunction. 2021 Aug 30. In: *StatPearls* [Internet]. Treasure Island (FL): StatPearls Publishing; 2021 Jan–.PMID: 32809578.

Yi S. Q., An J. X., Liao C. C., Lei S., Jin H., Tuo B. G. The role of corticotropin-releasing hormone (CRH) family in tumors. *Neoplasma.* 2021 Sep;68(5):907-916.

Zhang X., Lei B., Yuan Y., Zhang L., Hu L., Jin S., Kang B., Liao X., Sun W., Xu F., Zhong Y., Hu J., Qi H. Brain control of humoral immune responses amenable to behavioural modulation. *Nature.* 2020 May;581(7807):204-208.

Chapter 27

Humoral Factors

Alicja Ochenduszka, Dorota Bartusik-Aebisher[*] and David Aebisher
Medical College of The University of Rzeszów, Rzeszów, Poland

Abstract

There are many important humoral factors significantly contributing to the humoral response of the human body. The basic protection of the human body against pathogens attacking it from the outside consists in an intact cellular, but also humoral inflammatory system and specific immunity. Humoral immunity comes from specialized cells that are derived from the bone marrow. They are type B cells and their main function is to produce the most important antibodies that are released when the need arises. It is worth knowing how to increase immunity, especially in the winter season, when the weather and weather conditions favor the development of many viral and bacterial infections. We should not allow ourselves to reduce immunity and take care of ourselves.

Keywords: antigens, humoral factors, K cells, lymphocytes, N-acetylmuramic acid, N-acetylglucosamine

Humoral factors are factors transported through the circulatory system, more specifically through the blood. Together with mechanical and cellular factors, they form the first line of defense of non-specific immunity against microbes that try to infect our body. The main mechanical factors include the specific

---

[*] Corresponding Author's Email: dbartusikaebisher@ur.edu.pl.

In: The Biochemical Guide to Hormones
Editor: David Aebisher
ISBN: 979-8-88697-492-8

structure of the skin and the mucous membranes present. Cellular factors include macrophages and granulocytes that have feeding properties, and finally, humoral factors are proteins produced by the body, involved in the fight against pathogens. These include interferons, lysozyme and the complement system (Gammoh et al., 2017). The general name of the humoral response comes from the observation that the factor responsible for detecting an antigen and causing the cascade of attack reactions towards it is in the acellular fluid, i.e., blood plasma, or in the tissue fluid.

Antigens produced by B lymphocytes are responsible for the detection of antigens. Their main task is to attach to the antigen in a specific way, thanks to which they "mark" the targets to be eliminated by specialized effector mechanisms such as phlegm cells, complement system or K cells. a complex system of cells consisting of Th, B lymphocytes and antigen presenting cells is responsible for the production of the correct antibody to function. The above-mentioned cells are connected with each other by a dense and often very complicated network of relationships between them, so the lack of one factor may disturb the functioning of the entire system responsible for the body's immunity (Gammoh et al., 2017).

The humoral response belongs to the so-called specific immunity of the organism. It starts to work only after the activation of non-specific immunity, i.e., certain features of the organism aimed at initial defense against the pathogenic pathogen. It includes the specific structure of human skin or the sweat produced at a low pH, which is a lethal environment for some bacteria. If the initial barrier of the organism, which are the factors of non-specific immunity, fails, the system of action of humoral factors is activated, participating in the specific - humoral immunity (Kellam et al., 2020).

One of the factors that make up the humoral factors are interferons. It is the general name for proteins created and released by cells in the body in response to detected pathogens. They belong to the cytokines, which in turn are part of glycoproteins. Their name comes from the ability to integrate into the process of replication of viruses in the cells of the human body, but their functions also include the activation of NK cells and macrophages that make up the cells of the immune system, regulating antigen presentation to T lymphocytes, strengthening the immunity of healthy cells, uninfected and thanks to the above-mentioned function they inhibit the synthesis of viral proteins, which inhibits the process of multiplication of viral cells. In humans, 7 types of interferons, divided into 3 groups, have been detected, which, among other things, during production, cause muscle aches and fever. The general function of all interferons is to fight neoplastic lesions and be antiviral agents (Kellam et al., 2020).

Another component of the humoral factors is lysozyme. It is a protein with a mass of about 14 kDa, capable of breaking down peptidoglycan, which is part of the bacterial cell wall. A polypeptide chain of 129 amino acids builds the primary structure of lysozyme. It has an active site. These are amino acid residues located on glutamate 35 and aspartate 52. Relatively far apart, I am actually quite close in space. The main function of lysozyme as a mechanism of non-specific immune response is antibacterial activity by destroying the cell walls of bacterial pathogens. It is present in macrophages, granulocytes and monocytes, and more specifically in their granules and in the tissue fluid. This hydrolytic enzyme breaks down beta-1,4-glycosidic bonds between N-acetylmuramic acid moieties and N-acetylglucosamine. Due to the presence of an outer cell wall, gram-negative bacteria are much more resistant to the action of lysozyme than gram-positive bacteria that do not have a cell wall (Read et al., 2019).

The complement system is also important in fighting pathogens. It consists of a group of about 40 proteins which, by intensifying inflammatory reactions and promoting phagocytosis, take part in the fight against pathogenic microorganisms that have managed to penetrate into the human body. The initiation of the complement system is a cascade, which means that each factor activates the next one and the lack of one of them may disturb the functioning of the entire system. There are three types of complement system activation, which are classic, lectin and alternative activation. The former is influenced by immunoglobulins present on the surface of the pathogen during the junction of the antigen-antibody complex (Tsibulnikov et al., 2019). Classical activation of the complement system leads to bacteriolysis. The alternative route, which is a faster option, takes shape from the moment of the penetration of the microorganism to the infection and its stages in the subsequent operation are almost identical to the classical route. The last, third way is the lectin way. It works by combining sugar from the surface of the bacteria with a lectin that has the ability to bind mannose. Its further stages are analogous to the previous routes and lead to the inhibition of the pathogen's activity (Zimmermann et al., 2019).

There are many other equally important humoral factors significantly contributing to the humoral response of the human body, however, those mentioned above are some of the most important. The basic protection of the human body against pathogens attacking it from the outside consists in an intact cellular, but also humoral inflammatory system and specific immunity.

The primary barrier to inhibiting the action of pathogenic microorganisms are phagocytic cells, but if not for the title, humoral factors ensure their proper functioning by enabling migration towards, recognition, highly effective and efficient absorption and killing of invaders. Humoral immunity comes from specialized cells that are derived from the bone marrow. They are type B cells and their main function is to produce the most important antibodies that are released when the need arises. It can be concluded that there are so-called "Factories" in which immunoglobulins are created in the peripheral blood, which consecutively absorb intruders attacking the body. Therefore, it is worth knowing how to increase immunity, especially in the winter season, when the weather and weather conditions favor the development of many viral and bacterial infections. We should not allow ourselves to reduce immunity and take care of ourselves, including supplementing Vit. D, and others that cannot be produced by the body itself and must be provided, for example, with food or special supplements.

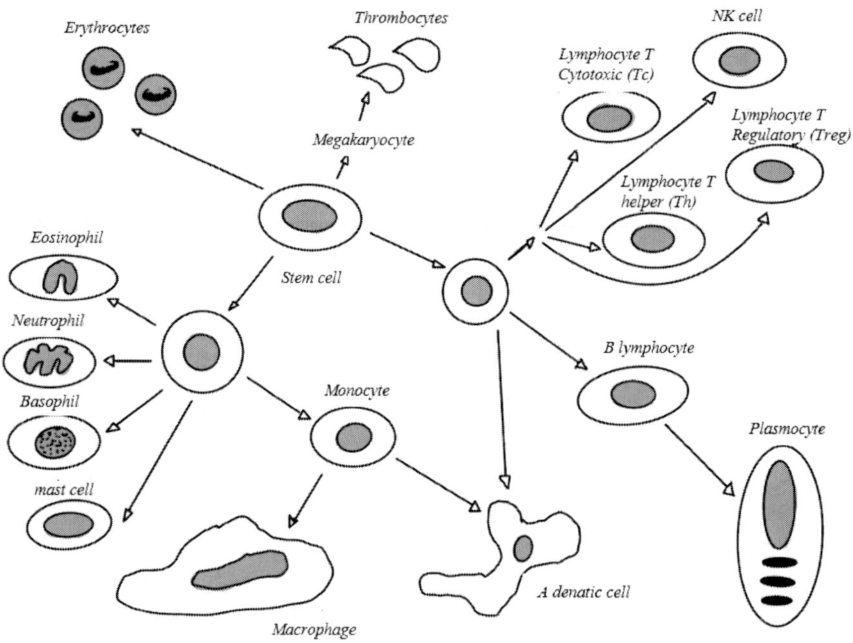

Figure 1. The figure shows the stages of the formation of cells involved in the humoral and cellular response of the human body.

References

Gammoh N Z, Rink L. Zinc in Infection and Inflammation. *Nutrients*. 2017 Jun 17;9(6): 624.

Kellam P, Barclay W. The dynamics of humoral immune responses following SARS- CoV-2 infection and the potential for reinfection. *J. Gen. Virol*. 2020 Aug;101(8):791-797.

Read S A, Obeid S, Ahlenstiel C, Ahlenstiel G. The Role of Zinc in Antiviral Immunity. *Adv Nutr*. 2019 Jul 1;10(4):696-710.

Tsibulnikov S Y, Maslov L N, Gorbunov A S, Voronkov N S, Boshchenko A A, Popov S V, Prokudina E S, Singh N, Downey J M. A Review of Humoral Factors in Remote Preconditioning of the Heart. *J. Cardiovasc. Pharmacol. Ther*. 2019 Sep;24(5):403-421.

Zimmermann P, Curtis N. Factors That Influence the Immune Response to Vaccination. *Clin. Microbiol. Rev*. 2019 Mar 13;32(2):e00084-18.

Chapter 28

Cortisol

Marta Sowińska, Dorota Bartusik-Aebisher*
and David Aebisher
Medical College of The University of Rzeszów, Poland

Abstract

Cortisol is a glucocorticoid hormone. Its production increases in stressful situations, thanks to which it owes its common name – the stress hormone. It is secreted by the banded layer of the adrenal cortex and is formed by one of the two chains of enzymatic transformations as a derivative of cholesterol. It performs many different functions in the body, mainly metabolic, contributing to the maintenance of homeostasis. The mechanism of cortisol secretion is based on the principle of negative feedback in the hypothalamic-pituitary-adrenal system. Both excess and deficiency of the stress hormone manifest themselves in serious health disorders. The therapy associated with cortisol supplementation is known and used, but it carries many undesirable effects.

Keywords: glucocorticosteroids, cortisol, hormone, 17-hydroxyprogesterone, 11-deoxycortisol, Addison's disease

The subject of the article is a chemical compound belonging to the group of steroid hormones – glucocorticosteroids – which is cortisol. Glucocorticosteroids were discovered in the early 1900s, while cortisol was not isolated until 1939. The production of cortisol takes place in greater

---

* Corresponding Author's Email: dbartusikaebisher@ur.edu.pl.

In: The Biochemical Guide to Hormones
Editor: David Aebisher
ISBN: 979-8-88697-492-8

amounts during stressful situations, which is why it is commonly called the stress hormone, and its secretion by the striated layer of the adrenal cortex has an impact on our daily functioning and behavior in various situations. The action of this hormone causes in the liver an increase in gluconeogenesis, hepatic glycogen synthesis and hepatic protein synthesis. In other tissues, cortisol increases protein catabolism, which is associated with an increase in the concentration of amino acids in the blood. In addition, the stress hormone causes a decrease in glucose consumption and transport by cells, as well as an increase in glycogenolysis and lipolysis. Due to the important role of cortisol for the human body, the article will be a kind of review that will describe the chemical structure of this hormone, the mechanism of cortisol action and its regulation, and the disorders that appear in it. In addition, the situation of cortisol deficiency and excess (in whom it can develop and how large it can be) and the problems that may arise from these conditions will be described. The article will also focus on cortisol-related hormone therapy (is it well known and in what cases is it applicable) (Adam et al., 2017).

As a steroid hormone, cortisol is made up of a cholesterol molecule. Like other glucocorticosteroids, it has twenty-one carbon atoms and its summarized formula is C21H30O5. The secretion of adrenal cortex hormones is regulated by the hypothalamus (by the production of corticoliberin) and the pituitary (by the production of corticotropin). The mechanism of cortisol formation in the hypothalamic-pituitary-adrenal system is regulated by negative feedback (cortisol deficiency stimulates the production of corticotropin and corticoliberin, while excess stress hormone inhibits their secretion). Synthetic cortisol derivatives work in a similar way, therefore long-term corticotherapy may cause adrenal insufficiency (Blair et al., 2017).

The stress hormone is produced by one of the two chains of enzymatic transformation reactions. In one of them, enzymes transform cholesterol into cortisol by intermediate products in the following order: cholesterol, pregnenolone, progesterone, 17-hydroxyprogesterone, 11-deoxycortisol, and cortisol. The second chain of transformations is similar, but due to the different order of the enzymes, an intermediate product between pregnenolone and 17-hydroxyprogesterone is 17-hydroxypregnenolone instead of progesterone. The enzymes involved in the formation of cortisol from cholesterol are: 20α-hydroxylase, 20-lyase, 22-lyase, 3β-hydroxysteridodehydrogenase, D5-isomerase, D4-isomerase, 17α-hydroxylase, 21-hydroxylase and 11β-hydroxylase. Due to the chain mechanism of cortisol formation and its regulation in the hypothalamic - pituitary - adrenal system, it is sensitive to any changes at any stage (Fogelman et al., 2018).

The production of cortisol is initiated by stressful situations, sleep deprivation, obesity, intense or prolonged aerobic exercise, depression, alcoholism, pregnancy, estrogen treatment and some disease entities. On the other hand, the inhibition of the secretion of the stress hormone is observed during relaxation, massage, during music therapy or laughter therapy. A decrease in cortisol levels can also be noticed during magnesium supplementation and when consuming Omega-3 fatty acids. Under normal conditions, the secretion of cortisol is diurnal and reaches the maximum level in the morning and the minimum level around midnight. The transport of the stress hormone is mainly due to the carrier protein - transcortin, which belongs to α2-globulins, and is to a lesser extent dependent on albumin. Under physiological conditions, 90-95% of this glucocorticoid is bound, while the remainder is so-called free cortisol, which only in this form can diffuse into target cells and exert biological effects (Iob et al., 2019).

Serious disturbances in cortisol secretion related to its deficiency are observed in people with adrenal insufficiency. Stress hormone deficiencies caused by such a condition are the cause of diseases such as chronic adrenal insufficiency, manifested in the form of Addison's disease (as the primary adrenal insufficiency caused by cortisol deficiency as a result of direct damage to the adrenal glands), or life-threatening adrenal crisis (caused by sudden, severe cortisol deficiency). Symptoms of cortisol deficiency may include: poor tolerance to stressful situations, easy fatigue, lower blood pressure or weight loss. On the other hand, adrenal tumors can overproduce cortisol, as is the case in Cushing's syndrome. The overproduction of the stress hormone may also be the result of hereditary syndromes such as the McCune-Albright syndrome or the glucocorticoid resistance syndrome. Excess production of cortisol is manifested by arterial hypertension, obesity, weakened immunity or osteoporosis. Hormone therapy with cortisol and its derivatives is known and used in the case of a deficiency of this hormone. It is often long-lasting and its aim is to normalize the concentration of cortisol depending on the time of day and stressful situations (increased dosing in the morning and when experiencing increased stress) (Kamin et al., 2017).

Cortisol is a hormone necessary for the proper functioning of the body. Its action is not local, but it covers all important systems in our body, which allows us to maintain internal homeostasis. The stress hormone also has a significant impact on mood changes, appropriate behavior in response to various stimuli (including, thanks to the preparation for stressful situations by enhancing the action of adrenaline and noradrenaline, for the fight-run reaction), pain sensation, body temperature, and food intake (due to the regulation of metabolic changes, mainly glucose and amino acids). Due to the fact that cortisol is necessary for the proper functioning of the body, its deficiencies have serious consequences. Therefore, a treatment based on supplementation with the stress hormone or its precursors is used. While glucocorticoid therapies like cortisol have many unwanted side effects, they are often the most effective treatment for many diseases. However, it should be remembered that, just like a deficiency, an excess of this hormone also carries an unfavorable effect, so its balanced concentration in the body is important. Further research into cortisol and stress hormone drug therapy could contribute to a better understanding of the mechanisms of action of this hormone and the development of hormone therapy with fewer side effects and better use of cortisol in various conditions.

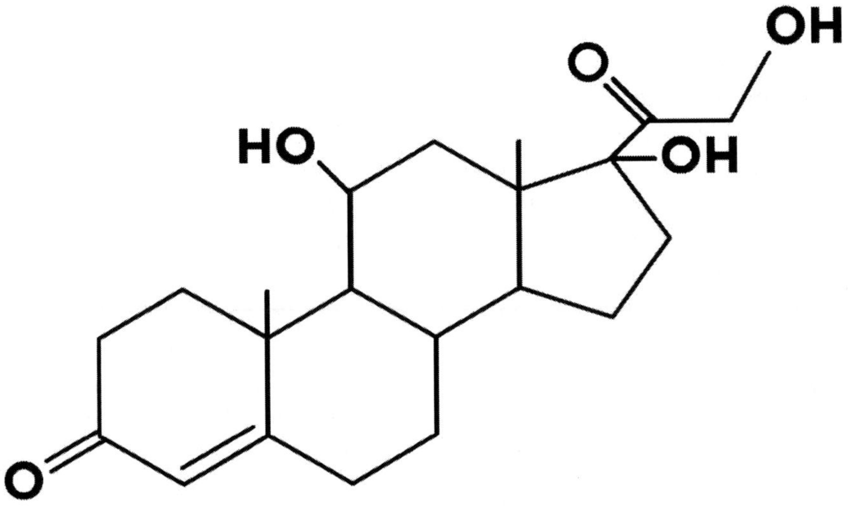

Figure 1. Structural formula of cortisol [Own elaboration].

References

Adam E K, Quinn M E, Tavernier R, McQuillan M T, Dahlke K A, Gilbert K E. Diurnal cortisol slopes and mental and physical health outcomes: A systematic review and meta-analysis. *Psychoneuroendocrinology*. 2017 Sep;83:25-41.

Blair J, Adaway J, Keevil B, Ross R. Salivary cortisol and cortisone in the clinical setting. *Curr. Opin. Endocrinol. Diabetes Obes.* 2017 Jun;24(3):161-168.

Fogelman N, Canli T. Early life stress and cortisol: A meta-analysis. *Horm. Behav.* 2018 Feb;98:63-76.

Iob E, Steptoe A. Cardiovascular Disease and Hair Cortisol: a Novel Biomarker of Chronic Stress. *Curr. Cardiol. Rep.* 2019 Aug 30;21(10):116.

Kamin HS, Kertes DA. Cortisol and DHEA in development and psychopathology. *Horm. Behav. 2017* Mar;89:69-85.

Chapter 29

Serotonin

Izabella Prządo, Dorota Bartusik-Aebisher*
and David Aebisher
Medical College of The University of Rzeszów, Rzeszów, Poland

Abstract

Serotonin is produced in the body by hydroxylation and decarboxylation of tryptophan, an essential amino acid – it must be constantly supplied in the diet. Foods rich in this compound are: fish (especially tuna and cod), milk, cheese, and pumpkin and other seeds, which is why a proper diet is so important for the proper functioning of the body. Serotonin is most concentrated in platelets and the gastrointestinal tract. It is responsible for the regulation of numerous biological processes such as: appetite, body temperature, blood pressure, and contraction of the bronchial muscles and blood vessels. The presence of serotonin is extremely important not only because of its regulation of mood, circadian rhythms, aggression, anxiety, but also it is responsible for smooth muscle contraction, proper body temperature, coagulation processes and proper blood flow due to pressure regulation.

Keywords: serotonin, 5-hydroxytryptamine, N-acetylserotonin, lysergic acid diethylamide (LSD), carcinoid tumors

In 1935. scientists obtained an extract from intestinal cells and considered adrenaline as a biogenic amine contained in it. Later studies proved that it was

---

* Corresponding Author's Email: dbartusikaebisher@ur.edu.pl.

In: The Biochemical Guide to Hormones
Editor: David Aebisher
ISBN: 979-8-88697-492-8

a previously unknown substance and called it enteramines, however, over time, its presence in blood serum was discovered and its name was changed to serotonin. It is both a tissue hormone and an important neurotransmitter in the central nervous system. Serotonin (5-hydroxytryptamine, 5-HT) is produced in the body by hydroxylation and decarboxylation of tryptophan, an essential amino acid – it must be constantly supplied in the diet. Serotonin is most concentrated in platelets and the gastrointestinal tract. It is responsible for the regulation of numerous biological processes such as: appetite, body temperature, blood pressure, and contraction of the bronchial muscles and blood vessels. It is also worth noting that its presence determines your well-being and feeling happy, hence it is colloquially called the happiness hormone. Its increased level in the body may reduce aggression and alleviate impulsive behavior, while its deficit is considered the basis of depression, therefore drugs based on increasing the level of this neurotransmitter are effective in their treatment. In the course of further changes in the pineal gland, serotonin is converted into melatonin, which also regulates the circadian rhythm. So, the role of serotonin in the body is endless, and that is what this chapter will be about (Bacqué-Cazenave et al., 2020).

Serotonin is produced as a result of enzymatic transformations, and more precisely, hydroxylation and decarboxylation of tryptophan in the brain's suture neurons in the midbrain, medulla and pons. The first step is the hydroxylation of tryptophan to 5-hydroxytryptophan, the enzyme in this reaction is tryptophan hydroxylase. The second stage leading to the formation of serotonin is the decarboxylation of 5-hydroxytryptophan in the presence of the enzyme 5-hydroxytryptophan decarboxylase. For the proper course of serotonin synthesis, an adequate content of vitamin B6, C and magnesium ions in the body is required (De Deurwaerdère et al., 2020).

As an important neurotransmitter, serotonin acts on many receptors, which are called serotonin receptors. They are found mainly in the cell membrane of neurons and, for example, in smooth muscle cells. Their main group are 5-hydroxy-tryptamine (5-HT) metabotropic receptors, whose task is to regulate ion channels in the cell membrane. Overall, 5-HT1 receptors are inhibitory, while others are stimulating. 5-HT3 receptors are an exception because they belong to the group of ionotropic receptors – their activation opens channels for Ca2 + and Na + ions, which causes depolarization and excitation of the neuron. Serotonergic receptors are involved in regulating many vital functions, such as food intake, intestinal peristalsis, depolarization and contraction of the muscle cell, and are involved in respiration and the regulation of heart function. Table 1 shows the most important serotonergic receptors, their location and function (Fouquet et al., 2019).

Table 1. Most important serotonergic receptors with their location and functions

Receptor type	Arrangement	Function
5-HT1A	Brain cortex, hippocampus, nuclei	Lowering cellular cAMP levels through G proteins
5-HT1B	Vascular smooth muscles	Blockage of the ganglion of the autonomic system, vasoconstriction
5-HT2A	Platelets, smooth muscles	Platelet aggregation, smooth muscle contraction
5-HT3	The digestive tract, the farthest field	vomiting
5-HT4	Digestive tract	Peristalsis of the digestive system, respiration processes

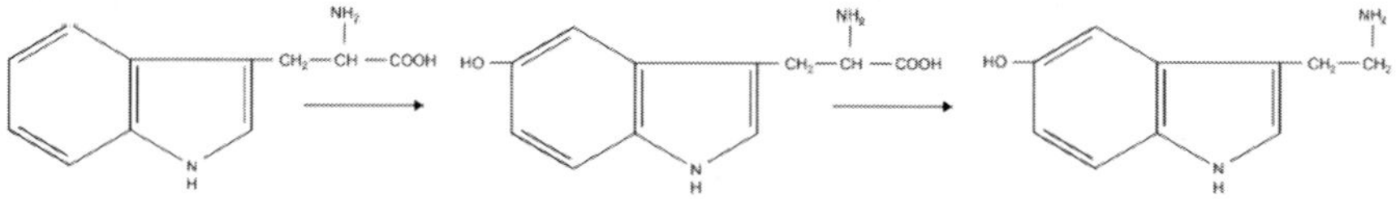

Figure 1. Serotonin synthesis pathway.

Serotonin as a neurotransmitter is directly related to anxiety, perceived mood and cognitive processes. It is also involved in the regulation of the circadian rhythm as it can be converted into N-acetylserotonin and then into melatonin, which is the main sleep hormone.

Moreover, an increased level of serotonin causes euphoria, and its deficiency causes depressive states, problems with concentration and insomnia. An example of substances that increase the level of serotonin in the body are hallucinogenic compounds such as, for example, lysergic acid diethylamide (LSD), which is its agonist. It binds to the 5-HT2 receptor, causing it to activate. Another example is 3,4-methylenedioxymethamphetamine, also known as MDMA, which, by binding to the aforementioned receptors, causes a feeling of fulfillment and happiness, but after a longer duration of action – irritability, deep sadness and anxiety. This is due to the increase in the level of serotonin released in the brain at the beginning of its action, and then depletion of its stores, as evidenced by the above-mentioned depressive states. The substances mentioned are addictive by causing the feeling of happiness. Carcinoid tumors, which are tumors that specialize in the production of this neurotransmitter, and a disorder called "serotonin syndrome," which results from taking various medications that affect the levels of 5-HT in the body, also affect the elevated levels of serotonin (Pawluski et al., 2019).

Serotonin deficiency is most often the result of a poor diet, and more specifically a lack of carbohydrates, which increase the level of serotonin, which is why people in a bad mood reach for snacks because it is associated with an improvement in their well-being. Low levels of folate, vitamins B6 and B12 will also reduce serotonin levels as they are essential for its synthesis. Too little serotonin causes aggression, sadness and insomnia. In people suffering from depression, the concentration of the main metabolite of serotonin, 5-HIAA, was found to be too low in the cerebrospinal fluid, and not, as it was once believed, too low a concentration of norepinephrine. Thanks to this discovery, drugs based mainly on inhibition of serotonin reuptake are used in the treatment of depression without affecting the reuptake of norepinephrine. Such drugs include: the tricyclic antidepressants – doxepin, venflaxine and fluoxetine. Moreover, in people with a mutation in the gene encoding the serotonin 2A receptor, the risk of committing suicide doubles as a result of a decrease in serotonin content (Stasi et al., 2019).

An appropriately high concentration of serotonin is determined by the appropriate amount of tryptophan, which must be supplied in the diet. Foods rich in this compound are: fish (especially tuna and cod), milk, cheese, and pumpkin and other seeds, which is why a proper diet is so important for the proper functioning of the body. However, it is worth remembering that it should be balanced, because addiction to temporary euphoric states as a result of eating products that increase the concentration of serotonin may lead to obesity and excessive overeating, which causes cardiovascular, respiratory and digestive diseases. The presence of serotonin is extremely important not only because of its regulation of mood, circadian rhythms, aggression, anxiety, but also it is responsible for smooth muscle contraction, proper body temperature, coagulation processes and proper blood flow due to pressure regulation. Its deficiencies are extremely harmful and can even lead to death as a result of mental ill health.

References

Bacqué-Cazenave J., Bharatiya R., Barrière G., Delbecque J. P., Bouguiyoud N., Di Giovanni G., Cattaert D., De Deurwaerdère P. Serotonin in Animal Cognition and Behavior. *Int J Mol Sci.* 2020;21(5):1649.

De Deurwaerdère P., Di Giovanni G. Serotonin in Health and Disease. *Int J Mol Sci.* 2020;21(10):3500.

Fouquet G., Coman T., Hermine O., Côté F. Serotonin, hematopoiesis and stem cells. *Pharmacol Res.* 2019;140:67-74.

Pawluski J. L., Li M., Lonstein J. S. Serotonin and motherhood: From molecules to mood. *Front Neuroendocrinol.* 2019;53:100742.

Stasi C., Sadalla S., Milani S. The Relationship Between the Serotonin Metabolism, Gut-Microbiota and the Gut-Brain Axis. *Curr Drug Metab.* 2019;20(8):646-655.

Chapter 30

Adrenaline

**Anna Wolan, Dorota Bartusik-Aebisher*
and David Aebisher**
Medical College of The University of Rzeszów, Rzeszów, Poland

Abstract

Adrenaline is essential for the proper functioning of the body. Thanks for action, the human body quickly evokes the necessary reactions, such as an increase in blood pressure or bronchial vacuum. In the first moments, in the situation of increased exploration of stress factors, adrenaline is released, followed by cortisol, which enhances the effect of adrenaline, thanks to which the body can cope with the stressor better and faster. Epinephrine increases the body's need for oxygen, increases body temperature and, together with cortisol, increases blood glucose levels to provide the body with the energy it needs. Adrenaline is called the fighting hormone for a reason, its action is quick and short-lived. Nowadays, where everyone is surrounded by many stressful and carcinogenic factors, epinephrine accompanies and mobilizes us every day, and each of us unconsciously feels many of its effects.

Keywords: adrenaline, catecholamines, N-methyltransferase, Parkinson's disease, epinephrine

Adrenaline, according to its international name, also epinephrine is an organic compound, a hormone and a catecholamine neurotransmitter. It is also referred

---

* Corresponding Author's Email: dbartusikaebisher@ur.edu.pl.

In: The Biochemical Guide to Hormones
Editor: David Aebisher
ISBN: 979-8-88697-492-8

to as the 3xF hormone (fright, fight and flight), i.e., the hormone of fear, fight and flight. It is a weak base with a melting point of 212 ° C, well soluble in acids with which it forms salts, and slightly soluble in water (Finn et al., 2020). For the first time, a Polish physiologist, Napoleon Cybulski, who in 1895, together with Władysław Szymonowicz, discovered the hormonal effect of the adrenal medulla, isolated adrenaline. Epinephrine is the first hormone obtained in a crystalline state in 1901 by the Japanese chemist Jokichi Takamine, and the artificial manufacturing process was developed in 1904 by Friedrich Stolz, a German chemist. It is a derivative of catechol, which is obtained in living organisms as a result of the reaction of two amino acids – phenylalanine and tyrosine. It is formed in pheochromocytoma in five stages, each of which is controlled by a specific enzyme and is stored in pheochromocytoma (Finn et al., 2020).

It has a sympathomimetic effect, i.e., it stimulates the sympathetic nervous system, which depends on the direct or indirect stimulation of the α1, α2, β1, β2, β3 adrenergic receptors, it stimulates the activation of α1, β1, β2 and β3 receptors, while the α2 receptors inhibit the cell. They are present in the central nervous system, where the α 1, α2, β1, β2 receptors are distributed and in internal organs, where the presence of receptors is more diverse; for example, β1 is present in the lung, β2 in the heart, and β3 in brown adipose tissue (Gough et al., 2018). Examples of actions on specific receptors:

- α1 - stimulate contraction of smooth muscles, thus increasing blood pressure;
- α2 - presynaptic receptor; inhibit the secretion of norepinephrine or other transmitters from the presynaptic end;
- β1 - have a positive inotropic and chronotropic effect;
- β2 - cause bronchodilation, contraction of arterial and venous vessels of the skin and mucous receptors;
- β3 - intensify lipolysis.

Adrenaline is released from the nerve endings of the sympathetic system and is produced by the endocrine glands originating from the nerve crest, i.e., the adrenal medulla, paragangular bodies, and C cells of the thyroid gland. The enzyme catalyzing the first stage of epinephrine synthesis is tyrosine hydroxylase, other proteins necessary for the synthesis are dopamine decarboxylase and β-hydroxylase, respectively. N-methyltransferase is responsible for the methylation of norepinephrine – thus the last stage of adrenaline formation (Gough et al., 2018). The release of catecholamines from the adrenal medulla is a consequence of stimulation of the sympathetic nervous system by stress stimuli, hypoglycemia, hypoxia, hunger, pain, fear, anger, and anger. Adrenaline levels drop during sleep. The action of epinephrine is based on direct stimulation of both α- and β-adrenergic receptors and is stimulating for the sympathetic nervous system. Contact of catecholamines with β receptors leads to the activation of adenylate cyclase and an increase in the concentration of cAMP in cells. A2 receptors are present on the presynaptic membrane, their activation reduces the content of cAMP, and stimulation of α1 receptors increases the concentration of IP3 and DAG in target cells (Rao et al., 2019). It plays an extremely important role in the stress mechanism in humans, its effect on the sympathetic system is manifested by the above-mentioned effect on the receptors and the broadly understood effect on the sympathetic system, manifested, for example, by bronchodilation, increase in blood pressure, inhibition of intestinal peristalsis. In a stressful situation, life threatening, fights, adrenaline increases the pain threshold and has a positive effect on physical and mental fitness. Its actions have the greatest impact on the circulatory system, the consequence of which is the acceleration of the heart rate, as well as the increase of its cardiac output through the mediated action of β1 adrenergic receptors (Rao et al., 2019).

The resistance vessels in some vascular beds, e.g., in the coronary circulation and in skeletal muscle, have β2 receptors that mediate vasodilation by adrenaline, which may sometimes lead to a slight reduction in peripheral vascular resistance, but always with an increase in arterial blood pressure. Adrenaline is an antagonist of insulin because it accelerates the process of glycogenolysis in the liver and muscles, gluconeogenesis in the liver and inhibits insulin-dependent uptake of glucose from the blood. This mechanism of action of adrenaline allows the maintenance of normal blood glucose levels and the supply of organs with the necessary glucose (Ring et al., 2018). It also has a significant impact on the body's lipid balance, as it supports lipolysis and the release of free fatty acids. Other actions of adrenaline affect the stimulation of metabolism and thermogenic processes at a specific time. Adrenaline is involved in hormonal changes by increasing the secretion of parathyroid hormone and calcitonin (Ring et al., 2018).

Thanks to its properties, adrenaline is used as a drug administered:

- intramuscularly
- intravenously

- subcutaneously

The most common way of administration is by intramuscular injection in the anterolateral aspect of the thigh. Said method is used in anaphylaxis, since adrenaline is classified as the drug of choice in the treatment of anaphylactic shock; raises blood pressure, relaxes the bronchi – facilitating breathing and reduces swelling around the mouth and face, eliminating the symptoms of acute allergies. There are no contraindications to administering epinephrine to a patient with symptoms of shock, it is the primary treatment of anaphylaxis, and delaying its administration may cause side effects. Epinephrine is used as the oldest effective drug in the treatment of bronchial asthma and asthmatic conditions (Regent et al., 2020). Due to its isotropic positive effect, it is used during cardiogenic shock and is used locally during ophthalmic and dental procedures to constrict blood vessels. Adrenaline is administered in low doses due to possible side effects, such as tachycardia or dilated pupils, which make it impossible to assess the central nervous system. There are also contraindications to the administration of epinephrine, which can include e.g., hyperthyroidism or arterial hypertension. The daily dose of the drug should not exceed 4 mg, and a single dose of 1 mg (Regent et al., 2020).

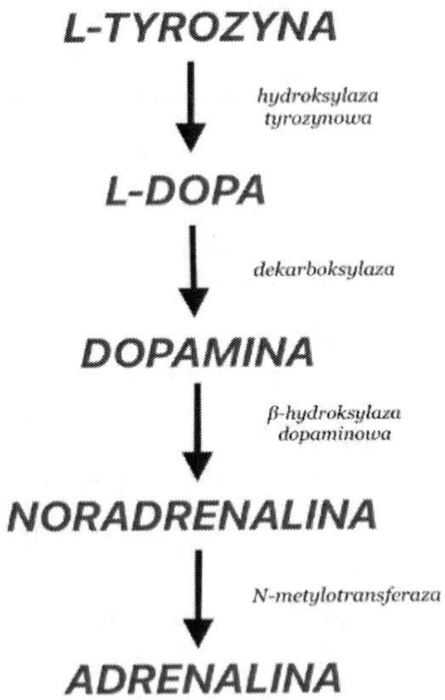

Figure 1. Scheme of adrenaline synthesis in cells of the adrenal medulla [Own elaboration].

Adrenaline is essential for the proper functioning of the body, it plays a key role in the stress mechanism and the body's immediate response to threats. Thanks to its action in the above-mentioned situations, the human body quickly evokes the necessary reactions, such as an increase in blood pressure or bronchial vacuum. It is commonly said that the release of adrenaline to the body carries only positive effects, however, long-term exposure to excessive action of epinephrine is associated with very negative consequences for health. In the first moments, in the situation of increased exploration of stress factors, adrenaline is released, followed by cortisol, which enhances the effect of adrenaline, thanks to which the body can cope with the stressor better and faster. Epinephrine increases the body's need for oxygen, increases body temperature and, together with cortisol, increases blood glucose levels to provide the body with the energy it needs. Chronic and constant stress also determines the production of adrenaline, which can cause e.g., stomach ulcers, constant increase in blood pressure, it also increases the risk of atherosclerosis, diabetes and Parkinson's disease.

Epinephrine is also the basic drug in anaphylactic shock, adrenaline in an ampoule should be obligatory for allergy sufferers, because the factors causing a rapid hypersensitivity reaction may be seriously life-threatening, e.g., due to a drop in blood pressure. Adrenaline is called the fighting hormone for a reason, its action is quick and short-lived. Nowadays, where everyone is surrounded by many stressful and carcinogenic factors, epinephrine accompanies and mobilizes us every day, and each of us unconsciously feels many of its effects.

References

Finn J, Jacobs I, Williams T A, Gates S, Perkins G D. Adrenaline and vasopressin for cardiac arrest. *Emergencias*. 2020 Abr;32(2):133-134. English, Spanish. PMID: 32125114.

Gough C J R, Nolan J P. The role of adrenaline in cardiopulmonary resuscitation. *Crit. Care*. 2018 May 29;22(1):139.

Rao Y. The First Hormone: Adrenaline. *Trends Endocrinol. Metab*. 2019 Jun;30(6):331-334.

Regent L, Johnson D. Adrenaline autoinjectors. *Clin. Exp. Allergy*. 2020 Jun;50(6):652-653.

Ring J, Klimek L, Worm M. Adrenaline in the Acute Treatment of Anaphylaxis. *Dtsch. Arztebl. Int*. 2018 Aug 6;115(31-32):528-534.

Chapter 31

Leukotrienes

**Wiktoria Mirowska, Dorota Bartusik-Aebisher*
and David Aebisher**
Medical College of The University of Rzeszów, Rzeszów, Poland

Abstract

The involvement of leukotrienes in inflammatory processes is the main factor that prompts scientists to conduct clinical trials to develop new anti-leukotriene drugs. So far, these drugs have been used in patients with mild, moderate and severe asthma as well as asthma with hypersensitivity to aspirin. They are also used in the case of nasal polyps, hypertrophic rhinitis and sinuses, urticaria, and digestive system diseases. In the future, anti-leukotriene drugs may appear in cardiology, and more specifically as an aid in the case of ischemia of tissues, including the heart muscle. Doctors place a lot of hope in them because they can contribute to the development of medicine.

Keywords: leukotrienes, T lymphocytes, erythrocytes, endothelial cells, vascular permeability, glucocorticosteroids

Leukotrienes are biologically active compounds, and their action is based on binding to the appropriate receptor. Their name comes from the words leukocyte and trien, and was introduced in 1979 by the Swedish biochemist Bengt Samuelsson. They are lipids closely related to the immune system – they participate in immune mechanisms and inflammatory processes.

---

* Corresponding Author's Email: dbartusikaebisher@ur.edu.pl.

In: The Biochemical Guide to Hormones
Editor: David Aebisher
ISBN: 979-8-88697-492-8

They are formed in the body from arachidonic acid, metabolized by:

- 5, 12, 15-lipoxygenase,
- cyclooxygenase.

Leukotrienes in their molecule have 4 double bonds. Sulfopeptide leukotrienes additionally have a cysteine group at the 6th carbon atom (hence their second name – cysteine leukotrienes) (Rubinstein et al., 2018).

The biosynthesis of these compounds in the cell requires the presence of the 5-lipoxidase enzyme and the FLAP protein as well as stimuli, which may become e.g., anti-IgE antibodies or phagocytosis and immune complexes. Leukotrienes can be found in cells derived from the bone marrow (the so-called primary cell sources of leukotrienes) – basophils, macrophages, eosinophils, basophils, mast cells, monocytes and neutrophils. Each type of cell differs in the number and type of leukotriene it produces. Additionally, secondary sources can be distinguished: endothelial cells, platelets, T lymphocytes, erythrocytes and the epithelium of the respiratory tract. During the production of leukotrienes, histamine is also often secreted, which supports inflammatory processes. Due to the fact that leukotrienes are rapidly metabolized, they cannot be stored, and their conductivity may be autocrine or paracrine (Sirois et al., 2019).

Leukotrienes, apart from prostaglandins and thromboxanes, belong to the group of physiologically and pharmacologically active compounds – eicosanoids, the source of which are 20-carbon polyunsaturated fatty acids (mainly the aforementioned archaquinodic acid). Arachidonate is formed from phosphatidyl diacylglycerols of plasma membranes by the action of phospholipase A2. First, leukotriene A-4 (LTA-4) is formed, which is metabolized to leukotriene B-4 (LTB-4) and leukotriene C-4 (LTC-4). The subsequent cleavage of glutamate and glycine produces leukotriene D-4 (LTD-4) and leukotriene E-4 (LTE-4). The C-4, D-4 and E-4 leukotrienes are called cysteinyl leukotrienes and are mainly produced by eosinophils and pulmonary mast cells, while the source of LTB-4 is activated neutrophils and alveolar macrophages (McGinty et al., 2020).

Leukotrienes perform many important functions in the human body. Among them we can distinguish:

- chemotactic properties for neutrophils, eosinophils and macrophages,

- activation of phospholipase A2 and influence on transport of Ca^{2+} ions,
- adherence to the endothelium in blood vessels and the possibility of penetration through it,
- stimulating the proliferation and release of cytokines in macrophages and lymphocytes,
- increasing the production of toxic oxygen metabolites.
- In addition, the discussed relationships affect specific systems. They are:

  – the circulatory system, where leukotrienes cause the constriction of blood vessels (leukotriene D4 has the greatest effect here) and the formation of a nettle blister together with redness.
  – immune system – the most important here is also leukotriene D4, enhancing the expression of interleukin-1 and, if necessary, replacing interleukin-2 in stimulating T lymphocytes to produce interferons. Together with leukotriene C4, it has the ability to modulate immune reactions, e.g., proliferation of fibroblasts and glomerular endothelial cells or dissemination of myeloma colonies in treated with CSF.
  – the respiratory system in which leukotrienes can cause bronchial smooth muscle contraction (in vitro studies have shown that they work 1000 times more than histamine in this case), stimulate their cells to grow, increase their overactivity and mucus secretion, reduce airway patency and damage the epithelium.

It is worth mentioning B4 leukotry, which is involved in the pathogenesis of diseases such as rheumatoid arthritis, gout or inflammatory diseases of the large intestine. It is responsible for chemotaxis, aggregation and adhesion of neutrophils to the vascular endothelium and the degranulation of these cells. It is also a factor in lowering the pain threshold for an inflammatory response (Jiang et al., 2018).

The presented situations are the effects of the actions of the discussed compounds that can be inhibited by appropriate mechanisms. They are, for example, inhibition of the activity of 5-lipoxygenase (5-LOX), inhibition of Lt synthetase or blocking LT-receptors. Due to the above division of mechanisms, we can distinguish appropriately separate groups of drugs, i.e., inhibitors of γ 5-lipoxygenase (e.g., Zileuton and Priprost, acting in the treatment of bronchial asthma, psoriasis, intestinal ulceration or hay fever), FLAP inhibitors, antagonists of the leukotriene receptor. B4, CysLT1 or CysLT2 receptor antagonists. There are also plant-derived anti-leukotriene substances such as betulin and betulinic acid. They are pentacyclic triterpenes, consisting of 30 carbon atoms and found in birch bark. They are able to inhibit the activity of the enzyme phospholipase A, which is necessary for the release of arachidonic acid from cell membranes and hence their anti-inflammatory action. Leukotrienes are of great importance in the course of cystic fibrosis, where there is an increased inflammatory response to respiratory tract infection. Their concentration in the secretions of patients is sufficient to induce a strong biological effect in the form of mucus production, vascular permeability, smooth muscle contraction and leukocyte chemotaxis (Tian et al., 2020).

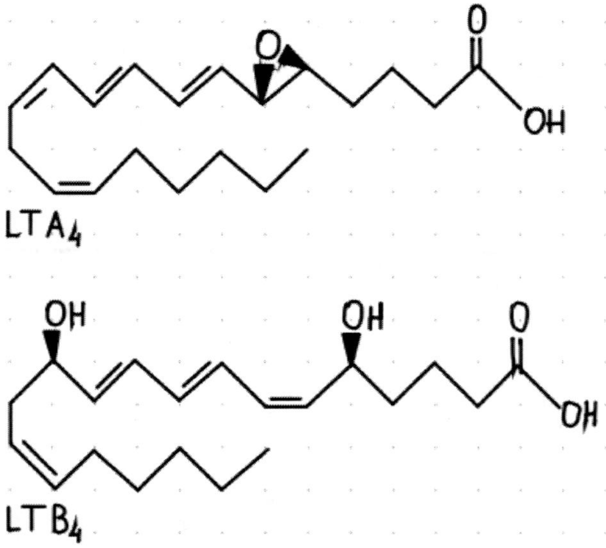

Figure 1. Formula of the leukotrienes LTA4 and LTB4.

The involvement of leukotrienes in inflammatory processes is the main factor that prompts scientists to conduct clinical trials to improve or develop new anti-leukotriene drugs. So far, these drugs have been used in patients with mild, moderate and severe asthma as well as asthma with hypersensitivity to aspirin. They reduce the dose of inhaled glucocorticosteroids and β-mimetics.

They are also used in the case of nasal polyps, hypertrophic rhinitis and sinuses, urticaria, and digestive system diseases (e.g., ulcerative enteritis). It is also possible to use them in the case of migraine or cancer, but this assumption is based only on preliminary clinical trials. Undoubtedly, they are related to pulmonology and treatment of patients with cystic fibrosis, while the mechanism of leukotriene activation and the source of their production have not been clearly defined. Given the complexity of the disease, the production of these mediators is probably a process activated by many coexisting mechanisms. In the future, anti-leukotriene drugs may appear in cardiology, and more specifically as an aid in the case of ischemia of tissues, including the heart muscle. Doctors place a lot of hope in them because they can contribute to the development of medicine.

References

Jiang X, Nicolls MR, Tian W, Rockson SG. Lymphatic Dysfunction, Leukotrienes, and Lymphedema. *Annu Rev Physiol,* 2018 Feb 10; 80:49-70.

McGinty JW, Ting HA, Billipp TE, Nadjsombati MS, Khan DM, Barrett NA, Liang HE, Matsumoto I, von Moltke J. Tuft-Cell-Derived Leukotrienes Drive Rapid Anti-helminth Immunity in the Small Intestine but Are Dispensable for Anti-protist Immunity. *Immunity,* 2020 Mar 17; 52(3):528-541.e7.

Rubinstein M, Dvash E. Leukotrienes and kidney diseases. *Curr Opin Nephrol Hypertens,* 2018 Jan; 27(1):42-48.

Sirois P. Leukotrienes: One step in our understanding of asthma. *Respir Investig,* 2019 Mar; 57(2):97-110.

Tian W, Jiang X, Kim D, Guan T, Nicolls MR, Rockson SG. Leukotrienes in Tumor-Associated Inflammation. *Front Pharmacol,* 2020 Aug 19; 11: 1289.

Chapter 32

Cholecystokinin

Aleksandra Wiechecka, Dorota Bartusik-Aebisher* and David Aebisher
Medical College of The University of Rzeszów, Rzeszów, Poland

Abstract

Cholecystokinin (CCK) is a peptide hormone that acts in both the digestive and central nervous systems.

It is responsible for the intake and digestion of food, therefore it plays an important role in the human body. CCK is structurally related to gastrin, and its CCK B receptors bind it. The role of this hormone in the central nervous system is diverse. It works not only to inhibit hunger, but also to reduce anxiety and panic attacks. A receptor antagonist by blocking the sites for CCK may protect against diseases such as stomach ulcers and anxiety. The diverse functions of cholecystokinin and its receptors arouse the interest of many scientists, which is why they take part in many studies.

Keywords: cholecystokinin (CCK), pancreatic enzymes, C-terminal amino acids, hormone

Cholecystokinin (CCK) is a peptide hormone composed of various amounts of amino acids, depending on the modification of its precursor. Its synthesis and secretion takes place in enteroendocrine cells in the duodenal mucosa and in the initial part of the jejunum.

---

* Corresponding Author's Email: dbartusikaebisher@ur.edu.pl.

In: The Biochemical Guide to Hormones
Editor: David Aebisher
ISBN: 979-8-88697-492-8

It was discovered in 1928 by Andrew Conway Ivy and Eric Oldberg (Ballaz et al., 2021). Since then, its various effects on the gastrointestinal tract and the central nervous system have been observed. Its main functions in the digestive system are:

- stimulation of the secretion of pancreatic enzymes;
- stimulation of contraction of the gallbladder;
- slowing down of gastric peristalsis;
- inhibiting the feeling of hunger;
- activation of visceral sensory nerves.

Thanks to the above-mentioned properties, cholecystokinin is responsible for the regulation of food intake, digestion and absorption of nutrients (Ballaz et al., 2021).

CCK is classified as a tissue hormone, i.e., it works only in the tissues that synthesize it. It is not transported with blood to distant tissues. Increased secretion of this hormone can be observed after eating meals high in protein and fats. Activation of cholecystokinin receptors causes the secretion into the duodenum of bile and pancreatic juice containing digestive enzymes such as lipases or amylases. The A-type receptor is mainly responsible for the feeling of satiety (Klingler et al., 2020).

In addition to regulating digestion and food intake in the small intestine, CCK is one of the most abundant neuropeptides in the brain. Its role is reduced to stimulating the satiety center in the hypothalamus, which inhibits the feeling of hunger. The cholecystokinin level test is performed in order to diagnose diseases of the pancreas and bile ducts (Klingler et al., 2020).

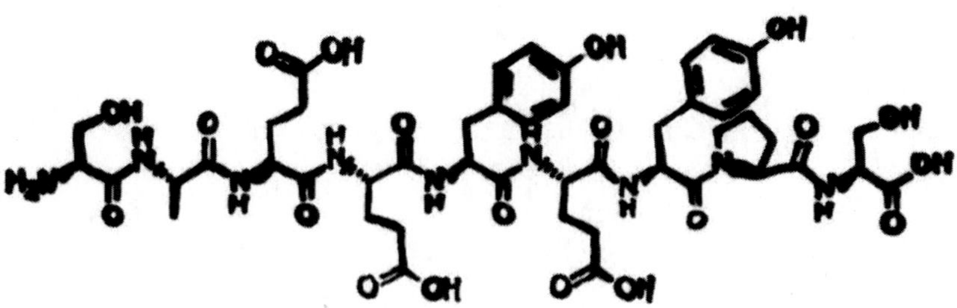

Figure 1. The structural formula of cholecystokinin.

Cholecystokinin belongs to the family of peptide hormones, which means that it is derived from amino acids. Its structure is similar to gastrin in that it has five of the same C-terminal amino acids. The precursor is preprocholecystokinin, the modification of which depends on the number of amino acids in CCK. Cholecystokinin has a short half-life. In most peptides in the chain, a sulfate group is attached to the tyrosine (Lach et al., 2018).

The increased release of cholecystokinin takes place with meals, especially those which are high in fatty acids and proteins. Its secretion is also controlled by the acetylcholine released from the vagus nerve. Its secretion is inhibited by somatostatin and pancreatic polypeptide.

The action of cholecystokinin on the digestive system is significant. It stimulates the follicular cells of the pancreas to secrete pancreatic juice, which contains enzymes that digest proteins, fats and carbohydrates. Its action causes an increased production of bile, but also its release into the duodenum through contraction of the gallbladder. The secreted bile supports digestion and absorption of fats into the body (Lach et al., 2018).

In the central nervous system, it is responsible, as previously mentioned, for suppressing the feeling of hunger. Receptors are distributed throughout the central nervous system. The greatest amount of cholecystokinin is found in the limbic system as CCK-8S. It also stimulates the vagus nerve, the antagonist of which is ghrelin with an inhibitory effect. Research has shown its association with anxiety and panic attacks, affecting the basal lateral amygdala, hypothalamus and hippocampus. Changes were observed in the cingulate gyrus, cerebellar worm, rampart, island and amygdala (Shen et al., 2019).

There are two types of cholecystokinin receptors – CCK A and CCK B. Most of the CCK A receptors are distributed in the digestive system. They are involved in the response to the meal. They are found in smaller amounts within the CNS. In contrast, cholecystokinin B receptors are found mainly in the central nervous system. They play a role in regulating satiety and anxiety. These receptors have been shown to be structurally identical to gastrin receptors. They can be found in selected areas of the digestive system. Both receptors are coupled with the G protein (GPCR), i.e., they are metabotropic, composed of seven transmembrane domains of a single polypeptide with the structure of α-helix, activating the G protein by neurotransmitters. Both receptors activate phospholipase C. The CCK A receptor also activates adenylate cyclase. It binds natural ligands and tyrosine with the attached sulfate group at the seventh residue from the C-terminus of the peptide leads to high binding affinity. Unlike the previous one, the CCK B receptor binds both the sulfate and non-sulfate forms with high affinity (Zeng et al., 2020).

The cholecystokinin receptor antagonist blocks the receptor sites for this hormone. Drugs should be selective for each receptor. Their action on CCK A protects against stomach ulcers or limits the development of gastrointestinal cancer. The receptors are involved in the suppression of anxiety to a lesser extent. More important, however, is the selective action of drugs on CCK B receptors. They are under constant research as their use in the treatment of anxiety, panic attacks and as painkillers is under consideration. CCK B also take part in the inhibition of gastric acid secretion (Zeng et al., 2020).

Cholecystokinin is currently the subject of much research. CCK-8 is being tested for its effect on reducing the size of meals consumed. This would make it possible to treat obesity and overweight in sick people.

Cholecystokinin is a peptide hormone that acts in both the digestive and central nervous systems. It is responsible for the intake and digestion of food, therefore it plays an important role in the human body. Particularly important in the consumption of foods high in protein and fats. Although it is secreted in the duodenum, it regulates the work of nearby organs, such as the secretion of pancreatic juice from the pancreas, bile from the gall bladder or slowing down the gastric peristalsis. CCK is structurally related to gastrin, and its CCK B receptors bind it. The role of this hormone in the central nervous system is diverse. It works not only to inhibit hunger, but also to reduce anxiety and panic attacks. Cholecystokinin receptors are G-protein coupled and their functions depend on the place of their occurrence. CCK A, found mainly in the digestive system, regulates digestive processes. The majority of CCK B receptors found in the CNS play a role in the regulation of satiety and anxiety. A receptor antagonist by blocking the sites for CCK may protect against diseases such as stomach ulcers and anxiety. The diverse functions of cholecystokinin and its receptors arouse the interest of many scientists, which is why they take part in many studies. This can help you fight overweight and obesity in the future.

References

Ballaz SJ, Bourin M. Cholecystokinin-Mediated Neuromodulation of Anxiety and Schizophrenia: A "Dimmer-Switch" Hypothesis. *Curr Neuropharmacol*, 2021; 19(7): 925-938.

Klingler M, Hörmann AA, Guggenberg EV. Cholecystokinin-2 Receptor Targeting with Radiolabeled Peptides: Current Status and Future Directions. *Curr Med Chem*, 2020; 27(41): 7112-7132.

Lach G, Schellekens H, Dinan TG, Cryan JF. Anxiety, Depression, and the Microbiome: A Role for Gut Peptides. *Neurotherapeutics,* 2018; 15(1): 36-59.

Shen CJ, Zheng D, Li KX, Yang JM, Pan HQ, Yu XD, Fu JY, Zhu Y, Sun QX, Tang MY, Zhang Y, Sun P, Xie Y, Duan S, Hu H, Li XM. Cannabinoid CB₁ receptors in the amygdalar cholecystokinin glutamatergic afferents to nucleus accumbens modulate depressive-like behavior. *Nat Med*, 2019; 25(2): 337-349.

Zeng Q, Ou L, Wang W, Guo DY. Gastrin, Cholecystokinin, Signaling, and Biological Activities in Cellular Processes. *Front Endocrinol*, (Lausanne). 2020; 11: 112.

Chapter 33

Hepcidin

**Natalia Ziaja, Dorota Bartusik-Aebisher*
and David Aebisher**
Medical College of The University of Rzeszów, Rzeszów,Poland

Abstract

Hepcidin is a protein hormone, determines the proper iron metabolism and the availability of this metal in the body. Thanks to its detection, it became possible to link mechanisms related to inflammation and anemia. It has been shown that too much iron in the brain, associated with hepcidin deficiency, may contribute to the occurrence of degenerative diseases such as Parkinson's disease, Alzheimer's disease, Huntington's disease. Lack of iron ($Fe3+$) leads to pathological deposition of deposits in the organs, which results in the occurrence of neurological disorders. Research shows that an increase in hepcidin in the brain regulates the expression of iron transporting protein in astrocytes, neurons and the blood-brain barrier.

Keywords: hepcidin, hormone, ceruloplasmin, hepcidin-ferroportin axis, Parkinson's disease, Alzheimer's disease, Huntington's disease

Hepcidin is a long-chain 25 amino acid peptide that is responsible for maintaining iron homeostasis in the body. It is mainly produced in liver cells, i.e., hepatocytes. Regulates the iron balance in the body. It causes the release of iron from macrophages and also inhibits the absorption of iron from the

* Corresponding Author's Email: dbartusikaebisher@ur.edu.pl.

In: The Biochemical Guide to Hormones
Editor: David Aebisher
ISBN: 979-8-88697-492-8

gastrointestinal tract. Inflammation or iron overload greatly stimulates the production of hepcidin by the liver cells. Hepcidin plays a key role in various types of anemia, e.g., inflammatory anemia. Then the concentration of hepcidin may increase up to 100 times. Its participation in kidney and heart diseases as well as obesity-related disorders is also observed. In addition, hepcidin belongs to the group of the so-called acute phase proteins, accompanies infections or neoplastic diseases. Mutations in the human hemochromatosis (HFE) gene lead to a deficiency of hepcidin or to its incorrect synthesis. This then leads to iron overload and contributes to the onset of haemochromatosis, caused by excessive iron absorption. Another genetic iron imbalance is iron resistant anemia. Then, the concentration of hepcidin in the blood serum increases, which prevents the flow and outflow of intracellular and extracellular iron (Agarwaet al., 2019). Understanding the mechanism of hepcidin's action and its role in blood and iron diseases may lead to the development of new therapies and the development of drugs that inhibit or enhance hepcidin transcription in in vitro models.

Iron is an important chemical element that is required in many biological processes. Both its deficiency and excess is equally toxic in the body. Therefore, it is necessary to maintain the iron balance, thanks to numerous regulatory mechanisms. This is possible due to the presence of hepcidin, a protein that regulates the concentration of iron in the plasma and thus controls the release of iron from the cells (Billesbølle et al., 2020).

The hepcidin (HAMP) gene is located on chromosome 19q13 and encodes preprohepcidin, consisting of 84 amino acids. Under the influence of convertases, prohepcidin is formed, consisting of 60 amino acids. On the other hand, under the influence of proteases, bioactive hepcidin is formed, consisting of 25 amino acids. The hepcidin receptor is ferroportin, which is an exporter of iron in the cell. After hepcidin binds to ferroportin, its tyrosine residues are phosphorylated, leading to its destruction in the lysosomes. At the cellular level, the IRP proteins are involved in regulating ferroportin expression, regulating iron turnover and the synthesis of proteins such as ferritin and TfR1. When the blood level of iron in the body is too high, hepcidin is produced, which inhibits the absorption and accumulation of iron. The HFE protein, transferrin receptor 1 and 2, bone morphogenetic protein 6, hemojuveline (HJV) and transferrin are involved in the process of transmitting the signal that stimulates hepcidin synthesis. Bone morphogenetic proteins (BMP) are also involved in expression and are involved in chondro-, neuro and osteogenesis (Ginzburg et al., 2019).

The protein BMP6 plays an important role in the regulation of hepcidin synthesis, as it acts autocrine or paracrine on cells. By binding to a receptor on the surface of the hepatic cell, it phosphorylates the signaling proteins SMAD1 / 5/8, which carry the signal to the cell nucleus. The complex then binds the SMAD4 protein and the hepcidin gene is transcribed in the nucleus.

Hepcidin expression depends on many factors and is influenced by:

- the state of iron economy
- erythropoietin (EPO)
- hypoxia
- inflammation

Erythropoietin (EPO) binds to a receptor (EPO-R) on the surface of liver cells and inhibits hepcidin expression. However, some researchers emphasize that EPO only indirectly affects the production of hepcidin, acting by increasing erythropoiesis in the bone marrow, which leads to a decrease in blood iron levels (Saneela et al., 2019).

In chronic inflammation, the concentration of hepcidin in the blood increases in order to reduce the concentration of iron in the blood and its availability to microorganisms. It is a type of non-specific defense reaction of the body. In chronic and acute inflammation, interleukin-6 (IL-6) increases hepcidin levels. It then stimulates erythropoiesis and inflammatory anemia in the presence of macrophages that are saturated with iron. The hepcidin-ferroportin axis is dysregulated in iron disorders. Too little hepcidin production leads to iron overload, which leads to the development of hereditary hemochromatosis and β-thalassemia. Hemochromatosis gene mutations accumulate excess iron by reducing the regulation of the BMP-SMAD signaling pathway in the liver or by developing resistance to hepcidin. In anemia such as β thalassemia, erythropoiesis releases erythropherron, which inhibits the release of hepcidin. When too much hepcidin is produced, iron is reduced and anemia develops, often seen in patients with chronic kidney disease. The hepcidin inhibitor (TMPRSS6) is mutated, which enhances the BMP-SMAD signaling pathway (Silvestri et al., 2019).

Hepcidin, which is a protein hormone, determines the proper iron metabolism and the availability of this metal in the body. Thanks to its detection, it became possible to link mechanisms related to inflammation and anemia. In inflammation, blood levels of hepcidin increased, which led to a decrease in iron levels.

It has been shown that too much iron in the brain, associated with hepcidin deficiency, may contribute to the occurrence of degenerative diseases such as Parkinson's disease, Alzheimer's disease, Huntington's disease. The conducted research showed that the excess of iron leads to the death of neurons in aceruloplasminemia and neuroferritinopathy. In the case of aceruloplasminemia, which is a genetic disease, there is a mutation in the ceruloplasmin gene. The lack of ceruloplasmin synthesis prevents the oxidation of Fe^{2+} to Fe^{3+}. Lack of iron (Fe^{3+}) leads to pathological deposition of deposits in the organs, which results in the occurrence of neurological disorders.

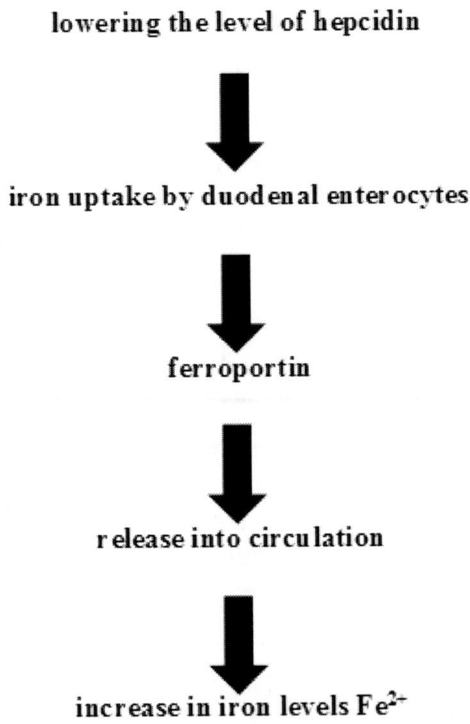

Figure 1. Mechanism of hepcidin's action in maintaining the body's iron balance

Therefore, the use of hepcidin may be of great importance in the selection of an appropriate therapeutic treatment of neurodegenerative disorders. Research shows that an increase in hepcidin in the brain regulates the expression of iron transporting protein in astrocytes, neurons and the blood-brain barrier.

References

Agarwal A K, Yee J. Hepcidin. *Adv. Chronic Kidney Dis*. 2019 Jul;26(4):298-305.

Billesbølle C B, Azumaya C M, Kretsch R C, Powers A S, Gonen S, Schneider S, Arvedson T, Dror R O, Cheng Y, Manglik A. Structure of hepcidin-bound ferroportin reveals iron homeostatic mechanisms. *Nature*. 2020 Oct;586(7831):807-811.

Ginzburg Y Z. Hepcidin-ferroportin axis in health and disease. *Vitam. Horm*. 2019;110:17-45.

Saneela S, Iqbal R, Raza A, Qamar M F. Hepcidin: A key regulator of iron. *J. Pak. Med. Assoc*. 2019 Aug;69(8):1170-1175. PMID: 31431773.

Silvestri L, Nai A, Dulja A, Pagani A. Hepcidin and the BMP-SMAD pathway: An unexpected liaison. *Vitam. Horm*. 2019;110:71-99.

Chapter 34

Prolactin

**Klaudia Dynarowicz, Dorota Bartusik-Aebisher*
and David Aebisher**
Medical College of The University of Rzeszów, Poland

Abstract

Prolactin is a protein hormone located in the anterior pituitary gland. Prolactin is a pleiotropic hormone with complex expression regulation. Lactotroph cells in the pituitary gland produce prolactin, where it is stored and then released into the bloodstream. It acts as a cytokine and plays an important role in human immune responses. It affects the metabolism, functions of the immune system and the functioning of the central nervous system. Due to its multitasking nature, the correct physiology of this hormone is extremely important.

Keywords: prolactin, lactotroph cells, hypothalamus, chronic stress, liver disease, hypothyroidism

Prolactin is a protein hormone located in the anterior pituitary gland. The pituitary gland sits directly behind the nasal bridge in a protective boney structure and it is connected to the hypothalamus by the infundibular stalk. The hypothalamus is largely responsible for regulating the synthesis and secretion of various hormones within the pituitary gland, including Prolactin. The pituitary gland is structurally divided into anterior and posterior regions.

* Corresponding Author's Email: dbartusikaebisher@ur.edu.pl.

In: The Biochemical Guide to Hormones
Editor: David Aebisher
ISBN: 979-8-88697-492-8

In humans, prolactin is produced both in the front portion of the pituitary gland (anterior pituitary gland) and in a range of sites elsewhere in the body. Its name comes from its key role in promoting milk production during lactation (Lopez-Vicchi, et al., 2020). It is a 200 amino acid peptide hormone (McMurray, 2001). Its main task is to stimulate the mammary glands to produce milk in the postpartùm period, inhibiting ovulation. Prolactin is a pleiotropic hormone with complex expression regulation (Cabrera-Reyes, et al., 2017). Lactotroph cells in the pituitary gland produce prolactin, where it is stored and then released into the bloodstream. Human prolactin is also produced in the uterus, immune cells, brain, breasts, prostate, skin and adipose tissue. Prolactin is also produced by lymphocytes and other immune cells. It acts as a cytokine and plays an important role in human immune responses. Prolactin effects on immunological systems may depend on concentration, resulting in immunostimulation at modest levels and inhibition at high levels. For example, in many cases of autoimmune diseases, the severity of the disease is lower or even remitted during pregnancy when serum prolactin level is elevated.

Chemically, prolactin exists in many post-translational forms, from size variants to chemical modifications such as phosphorylation or glycosylation. It is synthesized not only in the pituitary gland, as originally described, but also in the central nervous system, immune system, uterus and associated tissues of conception, and even in the mammary gland itself. Moreover, its biological activities are not limited to reproduction alone, as it has been shown to control various behaviors and even play a role in homeostasis.

It plays a significant role in breast physiology, especially in women. Its disappearance or increase in blood concentration indicates significant pathological changes / processes. The appropriate level of prolactin has a significant impact on the menstrual cycle of women. Recently, it has been confirmed that too high a level of prolactin leads to the disappearance of menstruation.

Prolactin as a single-chain polypeptide hormone was discovered in mammals in the 1930s. In humans, this hormone was described by Friesen in 1970 (Cabrera-Reyes, et al., 2017). Over the years, it has been shown that prolactin is not only related to the physiology of the mammary glands, but also has other functions. Prolactin stimulates the absorption of calcium in the intestines, strengthening the bone tissue. It also reduces the excretion of calcium through the kidneys (Charoenphandhu, Krishnamra, 2007). In some cases, it responds to stress. The proper level of prolactin in the blood is extremely important. Deviations from the norm (deficiency and its excess) may indicate mild or serious diseases.

There are times / conditions where the blood prolactin level rises naturally with no signs of disease or pathology. There is more prolactin in the body in such situations as: sleep, stress, increased physical activity, pregnancy, lactation or the postpartum period.

The natural physiological process in which the prolactin concentration increases is pregnancy and the period in which the woman is breastfeeding. Its concentration fluctuates significantly during this period. However, a long-term high prolactin level may indicate a number of pathological changes. Table 1 presents the diseases that cause the increased blood prolactin content.

Table 1. The reasons for the increased content of prolactin

Increased Prolactin - Causes
Taking medications for a long time, e.g. to lower blood pressure, antidepressants
Chronic renal failure
Chronic stress
Liver disease
Hypothyroidism
Pituitary gland adenoma

Prolactin is also responsible for the synthesis of cellular protein throughout the body. It has a luteotropic effect, stimulating the production of progesterone in the corpus luteum. It also supports the body's immune response. It stimulates the process of proliferation and differentiation of cells of the immune system, as well as angiogenesis processes. It also inhibits the process of multiplication of cancer cells, which is why it belongs to the group of anti-cancer hormones.

It also happens that the body produces an insufficient amount of prolactin. And we are dealing with a shortage of it. This condition is called hyperprolactinemia. However, it is extremely rare and affects people with hypopituitarism.

The list of prolactin properties is constantly expanding (Marano, Ben-Jonathan N, 2014). It affects the metabolism, functions of the immune system and the functioning of the central nervous system. Due to its multitasking nature, the correct physiology of this hormone is extremely important.

References

Charoenphandhu, N., Krishnamra, N. Prolactin is an important regulator of intestinal calcium transport. *Can J Physiol Pharmacol*. 2007, 85, 569-581.

Freeman, M.E., Kanyicska, B., Lerant, A., Nagy, G. Prolactin: structure, function, and regulation of secretion. *Physiol Rev*., 2000, 80, 1523-1631.

Lopez-Vicchi, F., De Winne, C., Brie, B., Sorianello, E., Ladyman, S.R., Becu-Villalobos, D. Metabolic functions of prolactin: physiological and pathological aspects. *J Neuroendocrinol*. 2020, 32.

Marano, R.J., Ben-Jonathan, N. Minireview: extrapituitary prolactin: an update on the distribution, regulation, and functions. *Mol Endocrinol.* 2014, 28, 622-633.

McMurray, R.W. Estrogen, prolactin, and autoimmunity: actions and interactions. *Int Immunopharmacol*. 2001, 1, 995-1008.

Chapter 35

Endocrine Disorders

Adamo Federica, Dorota Bartusik-Aebisher* and David Aebisher
Medical College of The University of Rzeszów, Rzeszów, Poland

Abstract

Endocrine disorders are a collection of conditions resulting from problems with a part of the endocrine system. This system uses glands throughout the body to produce and release hormones, which can affect a number of bodily processes. Endocrine disorders can be challenging to identify due to the range of symptoms they cause and their similarity to other conditions. However, people who are experiencing symptoms should contact a doctor, as the conditions typically require treatment.

Keywords: endocrine disorders, thyroid-stimulating hormone (TSH), adrenocorticotropic hormone

Endocrine disorders affect the endocrine system. This system uses glands throughout the body to produce and release hormones, which can affect a number of bodily processes. If hormone levels are too high or too low, or if the body does not respond to hormones correctly, a person may have an endocrine disorder (Borba et al., 2019).

---

* Corresponding Author's Email: dbartusikaebisher@ur.edu.pl.

In: The Biochemical Guide to Hormones
Editor: David Aebisher
ISBN: 979-8-88697-492-8

Endocrine disorders can result from:

- Dysfunction originating in the peripheral endocrine gland itself (primary disorders)
- Understimulation by the pituitary (secondary disorders)
- Overstimulation by the pituitary (secondary disorders)
- Rarely, because of abnormal tissue response to hormones (usually hypofunction).

The disorders can result in hormone overproduction (hyperfunction) or underproduction (hypofunction). Clinical manifestations of hypofunction disorders are often insidious and nonspecific (Hordon et al., 1991).

Hyperfunction of endocrine glands may result from overstimulation by the pituitary but is most commonly due to hyperplasia or neoplasia of the gland itself. In some cases, cancers from other tissues can produce hormones (ectopic hormone production).

Hormone excess also can result from exogenous hormone administration. In some cases, patients take hormones without telling the physician (factitious disease).

Tissue hypersensitivity to hormones can occur. Antibodies can stimulate peripheral endocrine glands, as occurs in hyperthyroidism of Graves disease. Disruption of a peripheral endocrine gland can rapidly release stored hormone (e.g., thyroid hormone release in subacute thyroiditis).

Enzyme defects in the synthesis of a peripheral endocrine hormone can result in overproduction of hormones proximal to the block. Finally, overproduction of a hormone can occur as an appropriate response to a disease state (Pal et al., 2020).

Hypofunction of an endocrine gland can result from understimulation by the pituitary. Hypofunction originating within the peripheral gland itself can result from congenital or acquired disorders (including autoimmune disorders, tumors, infections, vascular disorders, and toxins).

Genetic disorders causing hypofunction can result from deletion of a gene or by production of an abnormal hormone. A decrease in hormone production by the peripheral endocrine gland with a resulting increase in production of pituitary regulating hormone can lead to peripheral endocrine gland hyperplasia. For example, if synthesis of thyroid hormone is defective, thyroid-stimulating hormone (TSH) is produced in excessive amounts, causing goiter.

Several hormones require conversion to an active form after secretion from the peripheral endocrine gland. Certain disorders can block this step (e.g., renal disease can inhibit production of the active form of vitamin D). Antibodies to the circulating hormone or its receptor can block the ability of the hormone to bind to its receptor. Disease or drugs can cause increased rate of clearance of hormones. Circulating substances may also block the function of hormones. Abnormalities of the receptor or elsewhere in the peripheral endocrine tissue can also cause hypofunction.

Because symptoms of endocrine disorders can begin insidiously and may be nonspecific, clinical recognition is often delayed for months or years. For this reason, biochemical diagnosis is usually essential; it typically requires measuring blood levels of the peripheral endocrine hormone, the pituitary hormone, or both. Because most hormones have circadian rhythms, measurements need to be made at a prescribed time of day. Hormones that vary over short periods (e.g., luteinizing hormone) necessitate obtaining 3 or 4 values over 1 or 2 hours or using a pooled blood sample. Hormones with week-to-week variation (e.g., testosterone) necessitate obtaining separate values a week apart (Thakur et al., 2021).

Free or bioavailable hormone (i.e., hormone not bound to a specific binding hormone) is generally believed to be the active form. Free or bioavailable hormones are measured using equilibrium dialysis, ultrafiltration, or a solvent-extraction method to separate the free and albumin-bound hormone from the binding globulin. These methods can be expensive and time-consuming. Analog and competitive free hormone assays, although often used commercially, are not always accurate and should not be used (Thakur et al., 2021).

Free hormone levels can be estimated indirectly by assessing levels of the binding protein and using them to adjust levels of the total serum hormone. However, indirect methods are inaccurate if the binding capacity of the hormone-binding protein has been altered (e.g., by a disorder). In some cases, other indirect estimates are used. For example, because growth hormone (GH) has a short serum half-life and is difficult to detect in serum, serum insulin-like growth factor 1 (IGF-1), which is produced in response to GH, is often measured as an index of GH activity. Whether measurement of circulating hormone metabolites indicates the amount of bioavailable hormone is under investigation. Sometimes, instead of blood levels, urine (e.g., free cortisol when testing for Cushing disease) or salivary hormone levels may be used (Yalniz et al. 2020). In many cases, a dynamic test is necessary. Thus, in the case of hypofunctioning organs, a stimulation test (e.g., ACTH stimulation) can be used. In hyperfunction, a suppression test (e.g., dexamethasone suppression) can be used.

- Replacing deficient hormone
- Suppressing excessive hormone production

Hypofunction disorders are usually treated by replacement of the *peripheral* endocrine hormone regardless of whether the defect is primary or secondary (an exception is growth hormone, a pituitary hormone replacement used for pituitary dwarfism). If resistance to the hormone exists, drugs that reduce resistance can be used (e.g., metformin or thiazolidinediones for type 2 diabetes mellitus). Occasionally, a hormone-stimulating drug is used. Radiation therapy, surgery, and drugs that suppress hormone production are used to treat hyperfunction disorders. In some cases, a receptor antagonist is used (Yalniz et al., 2020). Hormones undergo many changes as a person ages.

- Most hormone levels decrease.
- Some hormone levels remain normal, including thyroid-stimulating hormone (TSH), adrenocorticotropic hormone (basal), thyroxine, cortisol (basal), 1,25-dihydroxycholecalciferol, insulin (sometimes increases), and estradiol (in men).
- Some hormone levels increase.

Hormones that increase, including adrenocorticotropic hormone (ACTH–increased response to corticotropin-releasing hormone), follicle-stimulating hormone, sex-hormone binding globulin, and activin (in men), gonadotropins (in women), epinephrine (in the oldest old), parathyroid hormone, norepinephrine, cholecystokinin, vasoactive intestinal peptide, vasopressin (also loss of circadian rhythm), and atrial natriuretic factor, are associated with either receptor defects or postreceptor defects, resulting in hypofunction.

Many age-related changes are similar to those in patients with hormone deficiency, leading to the hypothesis of a hormonal fountain of youth (i.e., speculation that some changes associated with aging can be reversed by the replacement of one or more deficient hormones). Some evidence suggests that replacing certain hormones in the elderly can improve functional outcomes (e.g., muscle strength, bone mineral density), but little evidence exists regarding effects on mortality. In some cases, replacing hormones may be harmful, as in estrogen replacement in some older women.

A competing theory is that the age-related decline in hormone levels represents a protective slowing down of cellular metabolism. This concept is based on the rate of living theory of aging (i.e., the faster the metabolic rate of an organism, the quicker it dies). This concept is seemingly supported by studies on the effects of dietary restriction. Restriction decreases levels of hormones that stimulate metabolism, thereby slowing metabolic rate; restriction also prolongs life in rodents (Yalniz et al., 2020).

Dehydroepiandrosterone (DHEA) and its sulfate levels decline dramatically with age. Despite optimism for the role of DHEA supplementation in older people, most controlled trials failed to show any major benefits. Pregnenolone is the precursor of all known steroid hormones. As with DHEA, its levels decline with age. Studies in the 1940s showed its safety and benefits in people with arthritis, but additional studies failed to show any beneficial effects on memory and muscle strength. Levels of growth hormone (GH) and its peripheral endocrine hormone (insulin-like growth factor 1 [IGF-1]) decline with age. GH replacement in older people sometimes increases muscle mass but does not increase muscle strength (although it may in malnourished people). Adverse effects (e.g., carpal tunnel syndrome, arthralgias, water retention) are very common. GH may have a role in the short-term treatment of some undernourished older patients, but in critically ill undernourished patients, GH increases mortality. Secretagogues that stimulate GH production in a more physiologic pattern may improve benefit and decrease risk. Levels of melatonin, a hormone produced by the pineal gland, also decline with aging. This decline may play an important role in the loss of circadian rhythms with aging. Estrogen replacement in older women is discussed under the treatment of menopause. Testosterone replacement in older men is discussed elsewhere. Endocrine disorders are a collection of conditions resulting from problems with a part of the endocrine system. This is a complex system that produces and distributes hormones throughout the body. These disorders occur when the endocrine system produces too much or too little of a hormone or if the body does not respond in the correct way to the hormone. Endocrine disorders can be challenging to identify due to the range of symptoms they cause and their similarity to other conditions. However, people who are experiencing symptoms should contact a doctor, as the conditions typically require treatment.

References

Borba VZC, Costa TL, Moreira CA, Boguszewski CL. MECHANISMS OF ENDOCRINE DISEASE: Sarcopenia in endocrine and non-endocrine disorders. *Eur J Endocrinol,* 2019; 180(5): R185-R199.

Hordon LD, Wright V. Endocrine disorders. *Curr Opin Rheumatol,* 1991; 3(1): 139-44.

Pal R, Bhadada SK. Managing common endocrine disorders amid COVID-19 pandemic. *Diabetes Metab Syndr,* 2020; 14(5): 767-771.

Thakur SS. Proteomics and its application in endocrine disorders. *Biochim Biophys Acta Proteins Proteom,* 2021; 1869(11): 140701.

Yalniz C, Morani AC, Waguespack SG, Elsayes KM. Imaging of Adrenal-Related Endocrine Disorders. *Radiol Clin North Am,* 2020; 58(6): 1099-1113.

Chapter 36

Endocrine System

Adamo Federica, Dorota Bartusik-Aebisher* and David Aebisher
Medical College of The University of Rzeszów, Rzeszów, Poland

Abstract

Endocrine system is indispensible for life in addition to the nervous system. Fundamental biological functions such as reproduction, growth, salt-water balance and emergency responses such as fight or flight are regulated to a fine tuning by the endocrine system in young and adulthood. Basically, the alteration in the above biological functions during aging is a consequence of altered hypothalamic-pituitary axes. Dietary restriction without malnutrition, physical exercise and nutraceutical interventions in elderly people reveal positive results in managing some of the endocrine disorders.

Keyword: hypothalamic-pituitary axis, steroids, endocrine system, adrenocorticotropic hormone (ACTH), thyrotropin-releasing hormone (TRH), growth hormone (GH), growth hormone-releasing hormone (GHRH)

The hormones created and released by the glands in your body's endocrine system control nearly all the processes in your body. These chemicals help coordinate your body's functions, from metabolism to growth and development, emotions, mood, sexual function and even sleep. The endocrine

* Corresponding Author's Email: dbartusikaebisher@ur.edu.pl.

In: The Biochemical Guide to Hormones
Editor: David Aebisher
ISBN: 979-8-88697-492-8

system coordinates functioning between different organs through hormones, which are chemicals released into the bloodstream from specific types of cells within endocrine (ductless) glands. Once in circulation, hormones affect function of the target tissues, which may be another endocrine gland or an end organ. Some hormones exert an effect on cells of the organ from which they were released (paracrine effect), some even on the same cell type (autocrine effect) (Borowska et al. 2018).

Hormones can be:

- Peptides of various sizes
- Steroids (derived from cholesterol)
- Amino acid derivatives

Hormones bind selectively to receptors located inside or on the surface of target cells. Receptors inside cells interact with hormones that regulate gene function (e.g., corticosteroids, vitamin D, thyroid hormone). Receptors on the cell surface bind with hormones that regulate enzyme activity or affect ion channels (e.g., growth hormone, thyrotropin-releasing hormone). Endocrine disorders result from disruptions of the endocrine glands and/or their target tissues (Baltaci et al. 2019).

Peripheral endocrine organ functions are controlled to varying degrees by pituitary hormones. Some functions (e.g., secretion of insulin by the pancreas, primarily controlled by the blood glucose level) are controlled to a minimal extent, whereas many (e.g., secretion of thyroid or gonadal hormones) are controlled to a great extent. Secretion of pituitary hormones is controlled by the hypothalamus. The interaction between the hypothalamus and pituitary (called the hypothalamic-pituitary axis) is a feedback control system. The hypothalamus receives input from virtually all other areas of the central nervous system and uses it to provide input to the pituitary. In response, the pituitary releases various hormones that stimulate certain endocrine glands throughout the body. Changes in circulating levels of hormones produced by these endocrine glands are detected by the hypothalamus, which then increases or decreases its stimulation of the pituitary to maintain homeostasis. The hypothalamus modulates the activities of the anterior and posterior lobes of the pituitary in different ways. Neurohormones synthesized in the hypothalamus reach the anterior pituitary (adenohypophysis) through a specialized portal vascular system and regulate synthesis and release of the 6 major peptide hormones of the anterior pituitary (see figure The pituitary and its target organs). These anterior pituitary hormones regulate peripheral endocrine glands (the thyroid, adrenals, and gonads) as well as growth and lactation. No direct neural connection exists between the hypothalamus and the anterior pituitary (Garcia-Reyero et al. 2018).

In contrast, the posterior pituitary (neurohypophysis) comprises axons originating from neuronal cell bodies located in the hypothalamus. These axons serve as storage sites for 2 peptide hormones, vasopressin (antidiuretic hormone) and oxytocin, synthesized in the hypothalamus; these hormones act in the periphery to regulate water balance, milk ejection, and uterine contraction. Virtually all hormones produced by the hypothalamus and the pituitary are released in a pulsatile fashion; periods of such release are interspersed with periods of inactivity. Some hormones (e.g., adrenocorticotropic hormone [ACTH], growth hormone, prolactin) have definite circadian rhythms; others (e.g., luteinizing hormone and follicle-stimulating hormone during the menstrual cycle) have month-long rhythms with superimposed circadian rhythms (Garcia-Reyero et al. 2018).

Thus far, 7 physiologically important hypothalamic neurohormones have been identified (see table Hypothalamic Neurohormones). Except for the biogenic amine dopamine, all are small peptides. Several are produced in the periphery as well as in the hypothalamus and function in local paracrine systems, especially in the gastrointestinal tract. Vasoactive intestinal peptide, which also stimulates the release of prolactin, is one. Neurohormones may control the release of multiple pituitary hormones. Regulation of most anterior pituitary hormones depends on stimulatory signals from the hypothalamus; the exception is prolactin, which is regulated by inhibitory stimuli. If the pituitary stalk (which connects the pituitary to the hypothalamus) is severed, prolactin release increases, whereas release of all other anterior pituitary hormones decreases. Many hypothalamic abnormalities (including tumors and encephalitis and other inflammatory lesions) can alter the release of hypothalamic neurohormones. Because neurohormones are synthesized in different centers within the hypothalamus, some disorders affect only one neuropeptide, whereas others affect several. The result can be undersecretion or oversecretion of neurohormones. Clinical syndromes that result from the ensuing pituitary hormone dysfunction (e.g., diabetes insipidus, acromegaly and, hypopituitarism) are discussed elsewhere (Malespin et al. 2019).

The cells of the anterior lobe (which constitutes 80% of the pituitary by weight) synthesize and release several hormones necessary for normal growth and development and also stimulate the activity of several target glands. ACTH is also known as corticotropin. Corticotropin-releasing hormone (CRH) is the primary stimulator of ACTH release, but vasopressin plays a role during stress. ACTH induces the adrenal cortex to release cortisol and several weak androgens, such as dehydroepiandrosterone. Circulating cortisol and corticosteroids inhibit the release of CRH and ACTH. The CRH-ACTH-cortisol axis is a central component of the response to stress. Without ACTH, the adrenal cortex atrophies and cortisol release virtually ceases. TSH regulates the structure and function of the thyroid gland and stimulates synthesis and release of thyroid hormones. TSH synthesis and release are stimulated by the hypothalamic hormone thyrotropin-releasing hormone (TRH) and suppressed (by negative feedback) by circulating thyroid hormones. LH and FSH control the production of the sex hormones. Synthesis and release of LH and FSH are stimulated mainly by gonadotropin-releasing hormone (GnRH) and suppressed by estrogen and testosterone. One factor controlling GnRH release is kisspeptin, a hypothalamic peptide that is triggered by increased leptin levels at puberty. Two gonadal hormones, activin and inhibin, affect only FSH; activin is stimulative, and inhibin is inhibitory.

In women, LH and FSH stimulate ovarian follicular development and ovulation. In men, FSH acts on Sertoli cells and is essential for spermatogenesis; LH acts on Leydig cells of the testes to stimulate testosterone biosynthesis. GH stimulates somatic growth and regulates metabolism. Growth hormone-releasing hormone (GHRH) is the major stimulator and somatostatin is the major inhibitor of the synthesis and release of GH. GH controls synthesis of insulin-like growth factor 1 (IGF-1, also called somatomedin-C), which largely controls growth. Although IGF-1 is produced by many tissues, the liver is the major source. A variant of IGF-1 is present in muscle, where it plays a role in enhancing muscle strength. It is less under control of GH than is the liver variant. The metabolic effects of GH are biphasic. GH initially exerts insulin-like effects, increasing glucose uptake in muscle and fat, stimulating amino acid uptake and protein synthesis in liver and muscle, and inhibiting lipolysis in adipose tissue. Several hours later, more profound anti-insulin-like metabolic effects occur. They include inhibition of glucose uptake and use, causing blood glucose and lipolysis to increase, which increases plasma free fatty acids. GH levels increase during fasting, maintaining blood glucose levels and mobilizing fat as an alternative metabolic fuel. Production of GH decreases with aging. Ghrelin, a hormone produced in the fundus of the stomach, promotes GH release from the pituitary, increases food intake, and improves memory (Poddar et al. 2017).

Prolactin is produced in cells called lactotrophs that constitute about 30% of the cells of the anterior pituitary. The pituitary doubles in size during pregnancy, largely because of hyperplasia and hypertrophy of lactotrophs. In humans, the major function of prolactin is stimulating milk production. Also, prolactin release occurs during sexual activity and stress. Prolactin may be a sensitive indicator of pituitary dysfunction; prolactin is the hormone most frequently produced in excess by pituitary tumors, and it may be one of the hormones to become deficient from infiltrative disease or tumor compression of the pituitary.

Several other hormones are produced by the anterior pituitary. These include pro-opiomelanocortin (POMC, which gives rise to ACTH), alpha- and beta-melanocyte-stimulating hormone (MSH), beta-lipotropin (β-LPH), the enkephalins, and the endorphins. POMC and MSH can cause hyperpigmentation of the skin and are only significant clinically in disorders in which ACTH levels are markedly elevated (e.g., Addison disease, Nelson syndrome). The function of β-LPH is unknown. Enkephalins and endorphins are endogenous opioids that bind to and activate opioid receptors throughout the CNS. The posterior pituitary releases vasopressin (argininevasopressin or antidiuretic hormone [ADH]) and oxytocin. Both hormones are released in response to neural impulses and have half-lives of about 10 minutes.

Vasopressin acts primarily to promote water conservation by the kidneys by increasing the permeability of the distal tubular epithelium to water. At high concentrations, vasopressin also causes vasoconstriction. Like aldosterone, vasopressin plays an important role in maintaining fluid homeostasis and vascular and cellular hydration. The main stimulus for vasopressin release is increased osmotic pressure of water in the body, which is sensed by osmoreceptors in the hypothalamus. The other major stimulus is volume depletion, which is sensed by baroreceptors in the left atrium, pulmonary veins, carotid sinus, and aortic arch, and then transmitted to the central nervous system through the vagus and glossopharyngeal nerves. Other stimulants for vasopressin release include pain, stress, emesis, hypoxia, exercise, hypoglycemia, cholinergic agonists, beta-blockers, angiotensin, and prostaglandins. Inhibitors of vasopressin release include alcohol, alpha-blockers, and glucocorticoids. A lack of vasopressin causes central diabetes insipidus. An inability of the kidneys to respond normally to vasopressin causes nephrogenic diabetes insipidus. Removal of the pituitary gland usually does not result in permanent diabetes insipidus because some of the remaining hypothalamic neurons produce small amounts of vasopressin. Copeptin is coproduced with vasopressin in the posterior pituitary. Measuring it may be useful in distinguishing the cause of hyponatremia (Poddar et al. 2017).

Oxytocin has 2 major targets:

- Myoepithelial cells of the breast, which surround the alveoli of the mammary gland
- Smooth muscle cells of the uterus

Suckling stimulates the production of oxytocin, which causes the myoepithelial cells to contract. This contraction causes milk to move from the alveoli to large sinuses for ejection (i.e., the milk letdown reflex of nursing mothers). Oxytocin stimulates contraction of uterine smooth muscle cells, and uterine sensitivity to oxytocin increases throughout pregnancy. However, plasma levels do not increase sharply during parturition, and the role of oxytocin in the initiation of labor is unclear. There is no recognized stimulus for oxytocin release in men, although men have extremely low levels.

Endocrine system is indispensible for life in addition to the nervous system. Fundamental biological functions such as reproduction, growth, salt-water balance and emergency responses such as fight or flight are regulated to a fine tuning by the endocrine system in young and adulthood. However, human beings during old age are deprived to some extent or fully of the above biological functions which may exhibit gender wise manifestations. Basically, the alteration in the above biological functions during aging is a consequence of altered hypothalamic-pituitary axes due to diminished hypothalamic responses to incoming downstream signals, diminished responses of the endocrine glands to the pituitary secretions and may be due to alterations of intracellular signaling players. Dietary restriction without malnutrition, physical exercise and nutraceutical interventions in elderly people reveal positive results in managing some of the endocrine disorders.

References

Baltaci AK, Mogulkoc R, Baltaci SB. Review: The role of zinc in the endocrine system. *Pak. J. Pharm. Sci.* 2019; 32(1): 231-239.

Borowska M, Czarnywojtek A, Sawicka-Gutaj N, Woliński K, Płazińska MT, Mikołajczak P, Ruchała M. The effects of cannabinoids on the endocrine system. *Endokrynol. Pol.* 2018; 69(6): 705-719.

Garcia-Reyero N. The clandestine organs of the endocrine system. *Gen. Comp. Endocrinol.* 2018; 257: 264-271.

Malespin M, Nassri A. Endocrine Diseases and the Liver: An Update. *Clin. Liver Dis.* 2019; 23(2): 233-246.

Poddar M, Chetty Y, Chetty VT. How does obesity affect the endocrine system? A narrative review. *Clin. Obes.* 2017; 7(3): 136-144.

Index

#

A

B

C

D

E

F

G

H

I

K

L

M

N

O

P

About the Editor

David Aebisher, PhD, DSc
Faculty of Medicine
University of Rzeszow
Rzeszów, Poland
Email: daebisher@ur.edu.pl